BITTER
MEDICINE

What I've Learned and Teach about
Malpractice Lawsuits (And How to Avoid Them)

RICHARD E. KESSLER M.D., F.A.C.S.
WITH PATRICK TRESE

Dedicated to the Memory

Of My Wife

Sheila Burke Kessler

TABLE OF CONTENTS

—

PREFACE

▬▬▬

I WANT TO REACH as many people as possible, so I decided to write this book in plain English and avoid technical jargon. I translated most medical terminology as I went along so readers with little or no medical vocabulary should be able to read straight through without looking things up. Some exotic words and phrases I didn't bother translating are there only to help the reader feel what it's like to be in a medical school, a hospital, an anatomy lab during a dissection, or an operating room during surgery.

I've recreated and dramatized situations in which I discuss actual clinical cases with students, patients, doctors and lawyers. For example: the telephone conversation reconstructed in the second chapter is typical of many I've had. It's not a verbatim account. But the specific details of the particular compartment syndrome case – and the tragic details of the other medical malpractice cases in this book – are dead-on accurate.

I've not identified the people involved by their real names and I've avoided identifying some specific geographical locations and institutions where things went seriously wrong. I see no benefit to be derived from re-opening old cases or old wounds. I've named only people who won't be harmed by having their names in print.

Thanks to lawyers who consulted me, I amassed a large file of the medical records I've reviewed. They proved to be effective teaching tools. Students, I've found, learn and retain more from studying medical disasters than perfectly executed procedures. Good outcomes, although important to study, tend to be predictable and happy endings can be boring for a student. Catastrophes are unforgettable.

To spare readers the ordeal of sitting through any of my real lectures or discussions, I've reconstructed and shortened some typical ones. I've also taken the liberty of creating composite characters to fill my labs and classrooms. The "real" students who endured my "real" lectures may be amused by the eloquence, erudition and wit displayed by their cranky old professor. They may also start wondering whether Socrates and his students were as eloquent in reality as Plato made them out to be. I hope mine will be happy to learn in what high regard I held them and how deeply I value all that they taught me.

I hope the stories I told my students will help readers make up their own minds about medical malpractice and what to do about it. Some Americans, for example, have been persuaded that many medical malpractice lawsuits are "frivolous" – or even that most are "without merit." If that were true, I would have had a hard time finding the cases I've presented to my students. But I did not. No deep research was required. I didn't have to go looking for horror stories. They came looking for me.

DEATH BY REMOTE CONTROL

"EVERYBODY'S HERE, DR. KESSLER."

"I believe you," I told the student standing at the conference room door. "But I'll just check to make sure."

I made a show of counting off the students with my finger. That got a few smiles from the seven young men and four young women seated around the long table in front of me.

"It's a good habit to develop," I said, not for the first time. "In the operating room, we count the surgical instruments, the sponges and the bandages going in to the OR and coming out so we don't leave anything inside the patient. In the classroom, I count the students. Remind me to count you again when you're leaving. I don't want somebody locked in here overnight with no way to get out."

That usually gets a laugh from the third-year medical students spending 12 weeks with me in my surgical practice at the VA hospital. This was Week Three and they were laughing more frequently now, which told me that they were absorbing what I was trying to teach them.

I walked to the blackboard. "The case we're going to discuss this afternoon involves a man with a bellyache. Anybody want to give him a name?"

"How about Alfred?"

"Okay, Alfred it is." I picked up the chalk, divided the blackboard into four columns: one for "Signs and Symptoms," one for "Lab/ Tests Results," one for the treatment my students thought the patient should receive, and one for the treatment he actually got. I wrote the patient's name in the first column and began adding what I knew about him.

"Alfred was a construction worker. Thirty-three years old. He was six-foot-three and weighed 235 pounds. He telephoned his family doctor at 1:50 a.m. That's ten minutes before two in the morning. Why? He had a 12-hour history of abdominal cramps, vomiting and diarrhea. I'm going to run down Alfred's case history and I don't want you to just sit there and listen. If you think you hear something inappropriate being done to or for Alfred, speak up. Interrupt me. Don't be shy. Stop the presentation and tell me what you think was wrong."

It was a new case for these students, but not for me. I've used this case for more than 15 years because it's a vivid example of how *not* to manage a case of acute abdominal pain – a dramatic lesson that students are not apt to forget. Whenever I reviewed this case, even the most reticent students became involved.

'Okay," I said. "It's about two in the morning. The family doctor listened to Alfred's description of his symptoms and made a diagnosis over the phone: viral gastroenteritis – that's influenza. Then he had Alfred admitted to the hospital – again by phone and . . . ." I stopped.

Eleven hands had shot up and everyone started talking at once. Some said that you can't diagnose acute abdominal pain over the phone. Others said that you have to see the patient and examine him. They all said that you have to put your hands on him.

"You're all absolutely right," I told them. "The family doctor had made his first mistake. And there were more to come. The doctor, who was still at home using the telephone, ordered a complete blood count and urinalysis," I paused. "Was that okay?" The students nodded and remained silent. But they were all leaning forward now. "The doctor also ordered intravenous fluids to be given at the rate of one liter every 12 hours." The hands shot up again. "That's not enough!"

"Why not?"

"Alfred's a big muscular guy doing hard labor," said one young woman. "He's like an athlete. He'll need 35-40 cc per kilogram per day."

"Yes," said another. "He'll need at least four quarts a day just to stay even with his basic water requirement,"

"He'll need more than that, if he's got a fever," said one of the young men.

"That's correct. Ordering one liter of IV fluids every 12 hours was the family doctor's second mistake. At that rate, Alfred's going to become dehydrated by at least two quarts of fluid per day." I paused to let that sink in. "Also, the doctor ordered an antibiotic – Ampicilin – to be added to each IV bottle." Again the hands shot up and I pointed to one of the students I hadn't called on before.

"Antibiotics are not effective for a viral gastroenteritis," she said. "And they are contraindicated in cases where there is undiagnosed abdominal pain."

"Why?" I asked the young man seated next to her.

"Because they can suppress an infection and mask the symptoms and delay the diagnosis."

"Right again," I said. "So the family doctor has made his third mistake. Now, as you can imagine, Alfred was very uncomfortable. So the doctor ordered Tylenol with a grain of codeine every 3-4 hours."

"Oh, stop!" One of the students almost rose from his chair. "Strong pain medication is contraindicated in a case like this." I asked him why and he answered quickly. "It can mask the symptoms and make diagnosing the problem more difficult than it already is."

"Correct. That was Mistake Number Four. And then the family doctor, who wanted Alfred to get some rest, ordered a barbiturate sleeping pill – Carbitol."

"Oh, come on," said one of my brighter students. "Is this a real case or are you just making it up?"

"Believe me, Guy. This really happened in a small rural community in the Midwest. And there's more. The doctor was told that Alfred had vomited so he ordered an anti-emetic – Compazine – to stop the nausea." The students looked at each other in disbelief.

"I see that you're all aware that Compazine is also a tranquilizer. So, at this point, the doctor had heavily sedated his patient with a narcotic, a barbiturate and a tranquilizer. That was his fifth mistake. And when he was told that Alfred was very thirsty, the doctor ordered clear liquids to drink." Up went the hands. They all knew that you should not feed a patient who has been vomiting. The stomach needs to rest. One student added that it was better to insert a nasogastric tube to stop the vomiting.

"Correct," I said. "It's the middle of the night. The doctor hasn't seen his patient yet and already he's made – how many mistakes?"

"Five," said one of the students. He checked his notes. "No, six!"

"And the doctor's still in his pajamas," I said. "But he finally got to the hospital. He saw Alfred at 8 o'clock that morning and asked him how he was feeling. What do you think Alfred told him?"

"He probably told the doctor that he was feeling much better."

"And, of course, he was," I said. "After all, Alfred had been loaded up with pain-killers and tranquilizers. He had slept most of the night and now he has less pain. Of course he feels better. But his temperature is 100 and his pulse is 100. His white blood count is 17,000 with a left shift. What's a left shift?"

"It's a term that means the number of white blood cells is increasing."

"And what does that indicate?"

"He's got an infection."

"Right on. Alfred's urine is concentrated with a specific gravity of 1035. What does that tell you?"

"He's dehydrated."

"Correct. I should also tell you that the doctor's physical examination of Alfred's abdomen revealed minimal tenderness on both lower quadrants. The doctor was not impressed. Is there any more information I can give you?"

"What did the CT scan or the ultrasound show?"

"Neither was available," I answered.

"Then what did the X-ray of the abdomen show?"

4

"No X-rays were taken until the next day."

"How were his electrolytes?"

"They were not measured for two more days."

"How about a surgical consult? He's had pain for 24 hours."

"A surgeon wasn't consulted for another two days."

The students were shaking their heads. "The doctor saw his patient again the next morning," I told them. "It's Day Two. Alfred's temperature is 101 and his pulse is 120. His abdomen is firm in both lower quadrants, his urine output is down and he's hiccoughing. The doctor is *beginning* to suspect a surgical problem. Alfred's white blood count is down to 12,000 but it's still showing a left shift."

"What did the X-ray show?" a student asked.

"It showed that the cecum was pushed over to the midline by a mass. But let me ask you this: why is Alfred's urine output down?"

"Because he's not getting enough fluids from the IV and he's dehydrated."

"Why is the white count down?" I asked.

"Because the infection is partially suppressed by the antibiotics."

"But why does Alfred have hiccoughs?"

That stumped them. Very few of my students can ever answer that question without a hint. "Could something be irritating the undersurface of Alfred's diaphragm?" One of the students made a guess. "Like pus, for example?"

"Right on," I said. "But the family doctor missed that. And he didn't see Alfred again until the next day, which was Day Three. By then, his patient's abdomen was distended. The tenderness and muscle guarding was maximum in the right lower quadrant. Alfred's temperature was 103 and his pulse was 120. His white blood count was back up to 17,000 and his potassium was low. So, what does the doctor do? He adds potassium to the IV and *finally* obtains a surgical consult. But the surgeon is not impressed with the physical findings and he procrastinates."

"The surgeon must be an idiot," one of the students said.

"Not necessarily. He may have been misled by the effect of the drugs on the physical findings. But what should the surgeon have done?"

"Operate?"

"No," I said. "He should have stopped the damn drugs and reevaluated the patient four to six hours later. Remember that: whenever you see a patient where the drugs may be masking the symptoms, *stop the drugs!* Wait and reevaluate!"

"So there was no exploratory operation?"

"Not until the next day – Day Four! By then, Alfred's abdomen was even more distended. He had a barium enema X-ray and that showed a defect in the cecum where the appendix was located. He was taken to the OR and explored, finally, and the surgeon found a ruptured appendix with pus everywhere in the abdomen. Alfred was critically ill and had developed septic shock." The students sensed what was coming.

"Alfred died the next day," I told them. "He left a widow and four children." The conference room was deadly quiet.

"Let me sum up: Alfred was a strong, healthy young man with a bellyache. He was diagnosed over the phone in the middle of the night. He went to the hospital and in four and a half days he was dead. We've found a series of mistakes that were made in his case, but there was one really big one. When Alfred's medical record was reviewed after his death, his chart contained 16 sets of doctor's orders and ten of them – *ten out of 16!* – were given over the telephone!"

I started gathering up my notes. "In the weeks to come, we'll be talking more about the correct way to handle cases of acute abdominal pain, but I want you to remember the biggest mistake that the doctor made in treating Alfred for what he assumed was causing his bellyache – and never, ever, try to practice medicine by remote control!"

I dismissed the class but the young men and women took their time collecting their books and note books. None of them seemed to want to leave the conference room. If I was finished with the day's discussion, they weren't. There was more they wanted to know about the case. (That's why I love teaching third-year medical students. They're bright and eager to learn.)

"What happened to Alfred's wife and children, Dr. Kessler?"

"Well," I said, "the widow got a lawyer and she sued the family doctor and the surgeon. The jury awarded her $250,000 which was a great deal of money for a small town. I'm told that, when summer came, the widow took a small portion of the settlement, bought an RV and took her children on a cross-country tour. That was something Alfred had promised his kids that he'd do for them someday."

"And you testified at the trial? Is that how you got the case material you presented today?"

"Yeah, I was an expert witness for the plaintiff. The widow's lawyer couldn't get any doctors in the area to testify against the two doctors who dropped the ball. So he had to get an outsider. That's what usually happens in small towns where everybody knows everybody. The trial was held in the dead of winter, a very cold, somber proceeding. I had to drive from the airport through a blizzard to get there."

They had more questions, of course. How did I feel about testifying against other doctors? What did I think about malpractice insurance and all those "frivolous lawsuits" people talk about? How did I get started testifying as an expert witness in the first place? I waved them off. "Some other day," I said to them. "Today, I don't want to talk about all that."

But I do now.

2

WHY NOW?

WHY WOULD A DOCTOR who has retired from the practice of medicine feel compelled to write a book about medical malpractice? Well, during the long, drawn-out debate about health care reform in the United States, I became sick and tired of the nonsense being spouted by a lot of politicians, pundits, preachers, lobbyists, advertisers, ax-grinders, and even doctors who should know better. There was hardly anyone who didn't have something to say about how to change – or resist changing – the way health care is delivered in the United States and every pontificator seemed to have an arsenal of anecdotes, urban legends, slogans, slanted statistics, misinformation, false claims, half-truths and even downright lies. No wonder patients and voters were baffled and confused. Frankly, I got fed up and felt an urgent need to offer a second opinion based on my own experience.

One book can't make such a dense fog bank of confusion evaporate, but I hope to poke a few holes in it. I feel obligated to tell you what I have seen, heard, experienced and learned first-hand over half-a-century as a medical student, an intern, a resident, a practicing physician, a general surgeon, an Army doctor, a teacher, a researcher and an expert witness in medical malpractice lawsuits.

Actually, that's not a bad place to start because too many Americans seem to believe anything they're told, whether it's true or not, if the voices they hear are loud enough and repetitive enough. So a lot of people now have strong beliefs about "frivolous lawsuits" instigated by "trial lawyers" who sue doctors and hospitals for "alleged malpractice." Spend an hour in a bar and you'll hear "on good authority" that most lawsuits filed against doctors and hospitals are without merit. You'll also hear that bleeding-heart jurors hand out millions of bucks to patients who suffer from nothing worse than bad luck. The voices are angry and full of conviction:

"We've got the best health care system in the whole world!" It may have been true, once upon a time, that the U.S. had the best health care system in the world, but that was 50 years ago. Today, at this writing, the World Health Organization puts the U.S. at 37 on its list. American citizens spend much more on health care than people in other modern, industrialized countries, but Americans get less health care for their money, higher rates of infant mortality and lower rates of life expectancy.

"We've got to cut down on all those frivolous lawsuits!" Really? Some recent reports suggest that about 100,000 Americans die each year because of medical errors. Could be more, could be less. But which of the malpractice lawsuits filed by the families of the deceased should be dismissed as "frivolous"?

"We need tort reform to rein in those unscrupulous trial lawyers and put caps on those ridiculous jury awards to their greedy clients!" Well, let's examine an actual medical malpractice case I reviewed. I dealt with an actual trial lawyer I'll call Kathleen, an attorney with a law firm for which I'd reviewed potential malpractice cases in the past. Kathleen wanted my opinion before she went ahead with a lawsuit. Did I think malpractice actually occurred? If so, did she have a case that would hold up in court?

WHY WAS THAT IMPORTANT for her to determine? She and her firm were working "on contingency." They would be paid if she won her case, but not if she lost. Besides not making any money, her firm would be stuck with the expense of pursuing the litigation. That averages out to $30,000. So taking on a case that was truly without merit and, therefore, truly frivolous, would be a foolish act. And Kathleen was no fool.

My involvement with her case began with a telephone conversation, typical of many I've had over the years. (I'm reconstructing it from memory and notes – not from a transcript.) I liked dealing with Kathleen. She had the curiosity and intelligence that mark a good no-nonsense lawyer, and she didn't waste time.

"We have a 15-year-old boy who had an operation for severe inflammation of the large bowel. You should see this kid, Dick. He's crippled for life."

I jotted the medical term "ulcerative colitis" on my yellow pad as she continued. "The inflammation was so severe that his entire large bowel had to be removed. Then the surgeon hooked up the small bowel to the boy's anus. He used a complicated intestinal pouch called a Parks pelvic ileal pouch. Are you familiar with that procedure?"

"I know what it is, but I've never used that kind of hook-up myself. So what happened?"

"After the operation, the boy developed 'severe compartment syndrome' in both legs. I'm not sure I understand exactly what that is."

"Well, you're not alone, Kathleen. Over the years, a lot of doctors have failed to recognize compartment syndrome in a timely fashion. All too often, the result's been a crippled or dead patient. Let me give you a quick anatomy lesson."

In the human body, I told her, there are four compartments in each leg, between the knee and the ankle. They are made up of dense, fibrous tissue called fascia. The muscles, nerves and blood vessels in a person's legs are enclosed in these compartments. If the pressure in a compartment becomes excessive, the contents of that compartment are threatened because pressure impairs the blood supply to the tissues in the compartment. That leads, first of all, to severe pain. As the condition worsens, there's a loss of muscle power. The patient won't be able to move his toes, for example. There will be a loss of nerve function that will cause paralysis and numbness or tingling in the feet and toes. If the pressure continues to increase, the major arteries will become blocked. That cuts off the supply of blood to the tissues in the compartment and all the tissues in the compartment will die. And that will cause severe, permanent disability.

"OK, I understand that," said Kathleen. "Pressure blocks the arteries, not enough blood gets to the compartment and that lack of blood kills all the tissues in the compartment. But what would cause the pressure?"

"There could be a lot of causes. Most fall into two major categories: inside pressure and outside pressure. If there's too much pressure from the outside, say, from something like a cast or a bandage that's too tight."

"The boy did have Ace bandages on his legs during his operation," said Kathleen.

"Well, they could have been wrapped too tightly. How long did the operation take?"

"About 16 hours."

"That's much too long, Kathleen! The average surgeon takes four to six hours for that procedure."

I asked where the operation was performed and how skilled the surgeon was. Kathleen told me that the surgery took place at the teaching hospital of a big medical school in the city where her law firm was located. I see no reason to name the city, the medical school's hospital or the surgeon. What's important to understand is that this was a well-respected hospital, that what happened really did happen and that the doctor was indeed experienced. He was Chairman of the hospital's Department of Surgery.

"What I don't understand," I said to Kathleen, "is why a surgeon with his credentials would take 16 hours for this procedure."

"This was the first time he'd ever performed this type of operation," she said.

"But he was assisted by a surgeon who had, right?"

"No, he wasn't. We thought that was rather peculiar."

"Peculiar? I'll say it was peculiar."

Actually, I thought it was downright arrogant, but I didn't say that out loud. I've never been too proud to ask someone to scrub in on a tough case when I thought I could use technical help. It's the right thing to do. All the man had to do was to get a surgeon to assist him who did have the experience he lacked. There's no shame in that; but this surgeon chose to go it alone. On my note pad, I wrote: *Why?*

"Didn't anybody say something to the surgeon about how long this operation was taking?"

"Not directly," she said. "We've learned that the anesthesiologist who was the attending on this case told his Chief of Anesthesia during the procedure that this boy was going to have trouble with his legs because they were being kept up in stirrups too long."

"And just how long were his legs elevated?"

"As far as we can tell, for most of the 16 hours."

"Well, there's your case, Kathleen. We're not supposed to keep a patient's legs elevated for more than a few hours. Keeping them up too long can definitely cause compartment syndrome."

"How, exactly?"

"As I said, the first major situation that can cause this syndrome is too much pressure from the outside – like tight Ace bandages. The second is increased pressure from inside the compartment – some condition that results in an accumulation of blood or fluid in a compartment such as interior bleeding caused by a broken bone."

"Our client wasn't bleeding in his legs."

"No, he wasn't. But his legs were kept elevated for most of the 16 hours. There's a reduction in blood flow to the legs when they're kept elevated too long. That causes tissue damage. When the legs are lowered at the end of a lengthy operation, the blood rushes into the tissues that have been ischemic – oxygen deprived. Fluid leaks out of the capillaries – the tiny blood vessels – into the adjacent tissue and that causes increased swelling in the compartment. I'm sure that was a major cause of this boy's problem. His problem would have been aggravated by the Ace bandages he was wearing – if they were too tight."

"Well, it sounds like we have a case," said Kathleen. "Anything else I can tell you?"

"There's something that still bothers me. I can't believe that the other people in the OR said nothing to the doctor. At least one of the nurses would have spoken up. They know that you can't keep a patient's legs elevated that long."

"Well, there's no record that any of the nurses said anything. So we can't tell if they did or not. And they sure aren't talking to us. Any idea why?"

"Fear of retaliation, maybe. My guess is they figure it's too dangerous to get on the wrong side of this particular department head. If I'm right, they won't volunteer any information, so you'll have to give them some protection and make them testify under oath. You might look into that."

"Oh, I will," said Kathleen. "There's something else you should know, Dick. We think the boy received too much IV fluid during the procedure. After surgery, his whole body blew up like a balloon."

"How much fluid did he get?"

"The record's not clear on that, but it shows he was 18 pounds heavier after his surgery than he was before."

"It's a wonder the poor kid didn't drown," I said. "That's another factor that helped cause his compartment syndrome, I'm sure. By the way, when did the hospital first become aware that the boy was having trouble with his legs?"

"Not until his mother brought it to their attention. Five hours after surgery, the boy still had a tube in his trachea. He couldn't talk, but he was able to write his mother a note that his legs hurt."

"And during those five hours nobody noticed something bad happening? A kid with a big incision in his belly starts complaining about pain in his legs as the anesthesia wears off? That should have set off an alarm bell."

"Well, it wasn't a very loud one. For the next two days there are numerous notes in the record by nurses, residents and attendings about the boy's leg pain, numbness, paralysis and severe pain on passive stretching of the muscles. But absolutely nothing was done for the boy."

"They should have taken him to the OR and done a fasciotomy to open up the compartments and remove blood, fluid and dead tissue."

"But they didn't," said Kathleen. "Not until two days later. That's four days after his operation. They finally asked for an orthopedic consultation. The orthopedists examined the boy and immediately diagnosed severe compartment syndrome in all four compartments in both legs and they recommended urgent surgery. They made that recommendation at 4:00 p.m. But the surgery didn't begin until after midnight – 12:30 a.m. to be exact. We think that was too long a delay in handling an urgent case. What do you think?"

"I agree. Time was of the essence. The sooner these cases are opened up, the better the result. The longer you wait, the greater the amount of dead muscle you'll need to remove. Is there anything else you want to tell me?"

"Isn't that enough?"

"It sure is," I said. "Do you want my opinion right now? Sue the bastards. That's my opinion."

"Well, that didn't take long," said Kathleen. "What kind of expert witnesses should I round up?"

"You'll need a pediatric or colorectal surgeon who's performed this operation. You'll also need an anesthesiologist because of the fluid overload and an orthopedic surgeon because of the delay in transporting the boy to the OR. Also, I'd like to examine the boy. I'm an anatomist as well as a surgeon; so I can give him a good orthopedic and neurological exam and tell you what muscles and nerves are no longer functioning."

"Okay, I'll have his parents make an appointment for him to see you. By the way, how many cases of compartment syndrome have you reviewed for law firms?"

"Four or five, I think. I reviewed the case of an 18-year-old who was shot in the leg and sustained a fracture of the fibula. The doctor didn't realize that there was internal bleeding in the boy's leg. By the time the doctor removed the cast, the boy's leg was gangrenous and had to be amputated above the knee. There was a compartment syndrome case I remember caused by the cast on a sprained ankle that was too tight. And another a boy who fractured two bones in his leg. That's three compartment syndrome cases off the top of my head."

"Did the cases have anything in common?"

"Yeah. In all of the cases I've reviewed, there were bad results because of procrastination and over-sedation with narcotics. In all the cases, the patients complained of pain, numbness, paralysis or severe pain when their muscles were stretched. In all those cases, their complaints were ignored until damage was severe. I was also struck by the ignorance about anatomy demonstrated in all four cases. If the doctors had learned their anatomy – or hadn't forgotten what they had learned – they wouldn't have made the mistakes they made."

"Did the cases you reviewed go to trial?"

"No, they all settled out of court. Your case will probably be settled too. Defense lawyers don't want jurors to hear about gross errors by highly-trained people who should have known better – especially when a kid's life has been ruined."

Kathleen worked quickly. A few hours after our phone conversation, the boy's parents called me for an appointment. Copies of the boy's medical records arrived in my office well in advance of his examination. The records, which I have kept in my files, backed up what Kathleen had told me about his initial surgery, as well as documenting what he had endured in the years that followed. I learned from the documents that he had undergone repeated procedures to remove dead tissue from both his legs, major skin grafting, tendon transfers to improve motion and also arthrodesis – obliteration of the ankle joint to correct deformity.

When the boy – now a young man of college age – arrived for his examination, he told me that his feet were always so numb that he was never sure where his toes were. Because of this loss of sensation, he couldn't tell if his shoes were fitting properly and so he would often develop ulcers on his toes and feet. The poor guy's legs were covered with unsightly scars and they were shriveled up from the loss of so many muscles.

I kept our conversation light and general, but it was obvious to me that his adult life would be tough. He would never be able to engage in any activity that required the vigorous use of his legs. He'd never be able to go dancing, play tennis or run to catch a bus. His normal activities – walking, squatting, climbing stairs – were difficult for him and they would become even more difficult as he grew older. Would I testify in his behalf? You're damn right, I would.

But I never got the chance. A few weeks after I examined the young man, Kathleen called to tell me that the medical malpractice suit had been settled out of court in favor of the young man and his parents for "a large, undisclosed amount," as they say in the papers.

"I'm happy for the family, of course," said Kathleen. "But, to tell you the truth, I was looking forward to a trial. The case put me in the mood for a good fight. How about you?"

"I'm sorry there won't be a trial," I said, "because now we'll never get any answers to the questions that are left hanging. Did the nurses tell the doctor something was going wrong or didn't they? Did anybody? And why did the doctor attempt a procedure he hadn't done before? Wasn't a more qualified surgeon available? Did the doctor have to operate himself? Or did he just want to? What can be done to prevent this kind of disaster from happening again? A trial might have given us the answers to a lot of questions. But we won't get them now; the doctor and the others in the OR that day can't be compelled to say any more than they've said already. So we'll never really know why the mistakes were made. We can only speculate."

"Well," said Kathleen, "there's a question I'd like answered. Can you tell me how some doctors become so arrogant or irresponsible that they can make such stupid mistakes? Care to speculate on that?"

"Speculate is all we can do," I told her. "I only know one thing for sure. They don't start out that way."

HOW DO I KNOW THAT? Almost without exception, the medical students I've taught over the years have been idealistic, hard working young men and women. Never have I met a medical student whose goal was to maim patients or kill them. I've flunked a few, but not because they were selfish or mean spirited.

On the contrary, they arrived at med school with the desire to help people and heal them and "do no harm." But there's an awful lot for medical students to learn and a lot to remember nowadays – a lot more than when I was starting out – and some kids just can't absorb that much specialized, scientific information no matter how hard they try. I hate to see them leave.

The young people who are able to continue on this rigorous course of study become more confident every year – and that's a good thing. It takes confidence to make a diagnosis and make a timely decision about a patient's need for treatment or surgery. But it takes a good deal of humility for a confident person to be able to say "I don't know" or "I need some help with this." Such humility is a virtue that's becoming increasingly important in this age of specialization and scientific breakthroughs.

Nowadays, one person can't know everything there is to know. Most young people who grow up to be practicing doctors, nurses or technicians realize that they are human and can make mistakes, that there's no shame in asking for information or help – if it's needed – and they do their best not to make mistakes.

Unfortunately, there are some medical students who gain too much confidence as they advance in their chosen profession – and not enough humility. They grow up to believe that they're infallible, that they're incapable of making a mistake. They over-estimate their own knowledge and skill and develop what they call "the courage of their convictions." Lesser beings call it "pride and arrogance."

It's a character flaw that often keeps doctors from recognizing that they are doing something wrong at the very moment they are making their serious – even crippling or fatal – errors. Some are unable to recognize that mistakes have been made, let alone that they are the ones who made them. So they can't learn from their mistakes and so they continue to make them – until they are somehow brought to their senses or stopped.

How do some doctors, who were once bright, motivated, idealistic young medical students wind up in situations in which they do cause harm – even great harm? What happens to them? Life happens to them, just as it does for everybody else.

Even the best medical education does not give anybody immunity from the Seven Deadly Sins that plague the rest of humanity. Nor does it automatically instill virtue. Skill in diagnosis and treatment – even compassion and a bit of wisdom – may come with practice. But infallibility? Never.

I don't believe that doctors make mistakes on purpose. Certainly, the doctor Kathleen sued did not intend to cripple the boy on his operating table; but cripple him, he did.

There are always plenty of people in a medical school's teaching hospital who could show him how to handle a boy's infected bowel efficiently and actually assist him in the OR. But this doctor couldn't or wouldn't admit to himself – or to others – that he might need a little help. For reasons that we'll never know, the doctor did not ask for help before performing an operation he'd never done before.

It was the doctor's misjudgment of his own ability that triggered the unfortunate chain of events. The operation took much longer than the doctor anticipated. Unable to stop the clock, he had to focus on keeping control of the procedure and reaching a good outcome.

Most likely, he was concentrating exclusively on the boy's open abdomen, not his elevated legs. If he had realized that keeping the boy's legs elevated for so many hours would cause compartment syndrome, he wouldn't have let it happen. But, obviously, he didn't know or didn't remember or didn't even notice. And, for whatever reason, none of his subordinates in the OR had the courage to warn the Boss that something wrong and dangerous was happening.

3

LEARNING FROM THE DEAD

▭

ON THE MORNING OF SEPTEMBER 11, 2001, I was in the anatomy laboratory deep in the basement of the New York University School of Medicine with two other professors and a score of cadavers which rested on cold metal examination tables, shrouded in waterproof white body bags with black trim. We were wondering why our students had failed to arrive.

A janitor burst through the door to tell us that America was under attack. We rushed upstairs to the main floor of the NYU Hospital to find out what was happening and to see if there was anything we could do to help. We joined the silent people crowded around the lobby TV sets. Like everyone else in the city, we were transfixed, staring at horror as it unfolded, listening for answers and reassurance.

One by one, the doctors, nurses, technicians and orderlies, whose shifts were ending or just starting, began moving away from the lobby and heading to their work areas. Like all the other medical people in Manhattan, we assumed that we'd be deluged with casualties. All over the city, doctors and nurses waited. But the flood never came. Ambulances eventually delivered a few injured people to the hospitals, but only a few. As the day lengthened, the truth sank in. The people in the towers had either escaped or were dead.

The sick and injured people who began to show up at the hospitals in the weeks and months and years that followed the attack were the heroic people who rushed to the World Trade Center to do what they could to help and who continue to suffer and die from what they were exposed to at Ground Zero.

If you lived below 14th Street in downtown Manhattan, as I did at the time, it was obvious that the air quality was extremely unhealthy. Whenever the autumn wind shifted to the north, Greenwich Village residents could tell that toxic fumes were emanating from the fires that smoldered and burned beneath the monstrous pile of rubble that had been the World Trade Center. The evidence was as plain as the ashes on apartment windowsills.

God only knew what was attacking the lungs of the men and women who were clearing the rubble and searching for human remains on what they called The Pile. EPA officials assured New Yorkers that the health of citizens working or living near Ground Zero was not in danger. But it was. That wasn't the first time the U.S. Government had lied, nor would it be the last. The America I grew up in had changed – perhaps forever.

SIX YEARS LATER, Osama bin Laden was still at-large and Americans were dying in Iraq as well as in Afghanistan. I was still teaching anatomy at NYU as a part-time, semi-retired professor handling the fall semester, grateful that my bright, young students had kept me from sinking into terminal pessimism.

Two weeks after the anniversary of 9/11 was observed at Ground Zero, I descended to the basement of the Coles Building, put on my white coat and walked through the two rooms containing 26 dead bodies. The students were just beginning to remove the wrappers from the cadavers, so I stood at the far end of the lab waiting for them to ask for help as they began their dissections.

I had noticed for several years that the majority of new medical students were now women. (When I was a medical student myself, there were only five females in my class of 100.) Also, I had observed the new first-year classes becoming more and more of an ethnic potpourri. No longer predominately white. The new students were black, brown, yellow and shades in between. There were young Christians, Jews, Muslims, and Hindus, plus a few atheists and agnostics, I'm sure. But all of them radiated so much eagerness that I wondered if they had any idea of what they were getting into.

The practice of medicine in America used to be fun when I was young. Doctors could spend time with their patients and decide the best course of treatment without being second-guessed or over-ruled by bureaucrats and business people. A lot had changed – and not for the better. I stood there, silently bemoaning the past, until a group of students asked me to give them some help with their dissections. I hurried over to their table. After all, that was what I was here for.

THE FOUR YOUNG STUDENTS would be studying the anatomy of the abdominal cavity for the next two weeks. The school's only information about their cadaver was that he was an 88-year-old male. They were to start by opening his abdomen and then chart a detailed exploration of the various organs they found within. But the students gathered around this cadaver were not sure how to begin because of a long vertical scar in the middle of the abdomen. And they couldn't identify a structure protruding through the abdominal wall in the upper right quadrant. I told them that asking for guidance was a correct decision.

"That scar tells us that this man had a major abdominal operation sometime in the past. You can tell because the incision went from top-to-bottom. But you won't know what was done until you get inside the belly.

"I know your dissection manual instructs you to take a scalpel and open the abdomen in the midline. But the scar tells you not to do that. Chances are you'll cut into several loops of bowel. They're probably stuck to the undersurface of the old incision by scar tissue called 'adhesions.' If you cut into the bowel, you'll have a shitty mess on your hands, pardon the pun."

The laughter broke the tension, which was what I wanted. The students were a bit less apprehensive. Even so, I decided to open up the cadaver's belly myself. "Watch what I'm doing," I told them. "I'm going to make an incision about one inch to the right of midline. By doing it that way, we'll have a better chance of avoiding the adhesions that may be present under the old scar."

"Before you start," one of the students said, "can you tell us what that thing is sticking out of the abdomen?"

"That's an ileostomy," I told them. "It's commonly referred to as a 'Rosebud' because it looks like one. It's really a segment of small bowel called *ileum* that has been brought out through the abdominal wall as a means of egress of intestinal content or urine. But we won't know which until we get inside.

"Fifty years ago, you'd know that a 'rosebud' in that location meant it was an ileostomy for expelling intestinal contents into a bag rather than the usual way. The diseased bowel was either by-passed or resected because of infection or cancer. But, for several decades now, urologists have been creating an artificial urinary bladder from a loop of small bowel.

"We won't know if this 'rosebud' is a new bladder until we sort out the continuity of the bowels and trace the transport of urine from the kidneys to the bladder. If this is a new bladder, it means that this man's original bladder was removed because of cancer.

"Unfortunately, we're not provided a medical history on these specimens, so we have to go in blind. I've been complaining about that lack of information for years. It shouldn't be hard to get a medical summary from the hospital or nursing home where the individual died. It'd sure help us here in the anatomy lab."

I picked up a scalpel and made a long incision. Once inside the abdomen, it became clear that there were adhesions everywhere. "See the loops of small bowel stuck to the undersurface of the old incision? And the loops of bowel stuck to each other? I'm going to have to take down all these adhesions with these curved scissors. It'll probably take about an hour. This is the kind of belly every surgeon dreads because the odds are very high that you can accidentally make some holes in the bowel,"

I began to dissect and separate the loops of intestines, slowly and carefully. The students watched my every move. After a while, a student asked, "What's your specialty, Dr. Kessler?"

"I'm a retired general surgeon," I said, without looking up.

"Were you a surgeon 50 years ago?"

"Fifty years ago, I'd just graduated from medical school."

"Which one?" a young women asked. "Oh, sorry! Does it bother you if we ask questions while you work?"

"Not at all. I went to McGill University in Montreal."

"You're Canadian?"

"No, an American. I went to McGill because it's a fine university. But the overriding reason McGill was my first choice? The tuition was only $600 per year."

A young man said, "Wow! We pay $28,000 a year. And that doesn't even include room and board or books!"

"Well, when I was applying back then, the tuition was $3,000 at med schools in the States. So I was real happy to be accepted by McGill."

"When was that?"

"1952 is when I started there. I graduated from Hobart College in 1951 – that's in Geneva, New York – but I couldn't get into med school right away. I applied to four med schools but they all turned me down." One young man said he'd applied to 15 schools; a young woman said she'd applied to 20. The students asked why I applied to only four schools.

"I could only afford four application fees," I told them "They were $25 apiece. The main reason I was turned down was my age. I was only 19 years old when I sent away for the applications and barely 20 when I went for the interviews. The med schools were giving preference to older guys, the World War II veterans. So I was advised to go to graduate school and re-apply in a year or two. That turned out to be the best advice I ever got. Changed my whole life."

And then I said, "Oops! I just got a hole in the small bowel! So I guess you'll have a chance to see how to suture bowels. Watch closely and, by the way, never say 'Oops' in the operating room, especially if the patient is awake."

Suturing the small bowel broke the monotony for a few moments. When I resumed the tedious task of separating all the remaining adherent loops of bowel, the students asked me what I found so special about graduate school.

"Well, I went to the University of Toronto where I was fortunate enough to spend a whole year studying anatomy with Dr. J.C. Boileau Grant."

"*The* Dr. Grant? The Dr. Grant of *Grant's Atlas of Anatomy?*"

"The very same," I said. "He was one of the greatest anatomists of the 20th Century, but I didn't know that at the time. He gave wonderful lectures, with marvelous drawings on the blackboard, but it took me about three months to understand everything he said because of his thick accent.

"He was a Scot from Edinburgh and he had been an army surgeon on the Western Front in World War I. He was a decorated war hero, a great mind and an extremely nice man. The year I spent with him proved invaluable to me when I became a general surgeon. And I'm sure it was his recommendation that got me into McGill University.

"As a matter of fact, that year at Toronto really paid off when I entered the medical school at McGill. I had already studied anatomy and histology, so McGill asked me to teach those two subjects to my classmates as a lab instructor. I learned ten times as much teaching those subjects than I had learned the year before."

As I continued the slow and somewhat tedious dissection, one of the students asked if McGill was the school that had a famous neurological institute. "Yes, indeed," I replied. "The Montreal Neurological Institute is probably the best in the world. It was founded by a famous neurosurgeon named Wilder Penfield. When we dissect the head and neck regions, you will learn about the nerve of Penfield."

"What was he like?"

"He was brilliant. He did magnificent research in mapping the various areas of the human brain. Actually, I shared a patient with Dr. Penfield when I was a second-year student."

"Come on, Dr. Kessler, second-year students don't have patients, do they?"

"Not as a rule, because they're still studying basic sciences like pathology and bacteriology. But, in my case, I was able to practice clinical medicine shortly after the beginning of my second year at McGill. I needed to generate some income to cover my room and board and I found an opening for an extern at Lachine General Hospital, a small hospital outside of Montreal.

"I got paid $50 per month plus room and board. In Quebec, an extern was a medical student who functioned just like an intern. We took all the histories on new admissions, started all the IVs, did emergency lab work, covered the ER sewing up lacerations and removing foreign bodies from people's eyes, assisted at emergency surgery – and even delivered babies when the doctor did not get there in time. I delivered about 30 babies at that little hospital. It was scary at first, but after one year, I was a pro.

"I remember one delivery, probably my first: a real shocker. The woman was a childless 42-year-old lady who wanted to have a baby but had stopped having periods. Her doctor had told her it was menopause. So she and her husband adopted a baby. Nine months later, she began to have abdominal pain and called her doctor. He told her to take two aspirins and call him in the morning.

"Two hours later, she called him back and told the doctor the pains were coming every ten minutes. He told her to take more aspirin and he would see her in the office in the morning. She called back an hour later and said the pains were terrible and coming every five minutes. The bells of enlightenment finally went off in her doctor's head. He told her to get to the hospital. He'd meet her in the obstetrical ward. She got there long before the doctor did.

"The OB nurse woke me at about 4 a.m. and told me there was a middle-aged lady in her unit with abdominal pain. She didn't know why the patient had been told to go to the OB unit. The nurse told me the woman didn't look pregnant. Her abdomen was hard. Could I come up and examine her? So I bounded up the one flight of stairs to the OB ward.

"By the time I got there, two tiny feet were emerging from the lady's vagina. It was a breech. We put a mask on the woman's face and put her to sleep with a gas whose name I can't remember after all of these years. The baby came out by itself and I just caught it. I tied off the umbilical cord, cut it, and went out into the hall to give the new father the good news. He passed out cold and I had to revive him with smelling salts.

"By now, the woman's doctor had arrived and when she came out of the anesthetic, we told her she had a baby boy who had red hair just like his momma. She insisted we put her on a gurney and wheel her out into the hall to hug her husband and telephone her mother and all of her girl friends."

One of the students asked what happened to the patient I shared with the famous Dr. Wilder Penfield.

"Oh, yeah, I got carried away there. Well, one night when I was the on-call duty extern, I was asked to see a 12-year-old girl in the ER who had a headache. It was about 11 P.M. But before I tell that story, I need one of you to hold the loop of bowel over to the right side. That'll help me take down these adhesions faster. Put on a pair of rubber gloves."

Once the student moved the loop of bowel out of the way, I was able to continue my dissection and my Penfield story.

"Even after all these years, I can still see that girl's face clearly. I even remember her name: Renata Heidersdorf. She'd been playing with a friend at the edge of a lake. They were pounding rocks with a hammer. A small piece of stone struck her on the left side of her nose, she said, under the corner of her eye. She felt a sudden, stinging pain, but after a few minutes she felt fine and went home. After supper, she became drowsy, developed a headache and vomited. Her parents also noticed her right eye was more prominent than her left eye.

"I thought her symptoms suggested an increase in intracranial pressure so I did a thorough neurological exam. I tested every cranial nerve, all her reflexes, her muscle power and her coordination. Everything was normal except for a slight droop of her right upper eyelid. And her right eye was, indeed, protruding out of its usual location. We call that *exophthalmus*. I saw a trickle of blood oozing out of each nostril and her nose was slightly tender.

"Her history did not make sense and I didn't have a clue as to what was wrong with this kid, so I had a technician take an X-ray of her skull. I was especially interested in a lateral view to see if she had a fracture of the nasal bone, but the X-ray was a blind stab in the dark. The technician said she saw something 'weird' on the X-ray film. I recognized the object. It was not a piece of stone. It was a 22-caliber bullet fired from some distance away.

"I called the Montreal Neurological Institute. They told me to bring the girl in and to keep her awake so they could do a neurological exam as soon as she arrived. I rode in the ambulance with the girl while her parents followed in their car. I had one hell of a time keeping her awake. I kept shaking her and calling her name. She did stay awake, but she managed to spray projectile vomit all over my clothes.

"We were met by Dr. Penfield and another fine neurosurgeon whose name was Cohen, I think. They took the same history I had taken and did a complete neurological exam which showed the same result as mine. Then we had a pow-wow and studied the X-ray. They told me it was critical to know the exact location of the bullet because it would determine which incision should be used.

"Dr. Penfield thought the bullet was in the orbit behind the girl's eyeball and Dr. Cohen thought it was in the infra-temporal *fossa* deep to the cheekbone or the Zygometic arch. Dr. Penfield turned to me and said, 'Dr. Kessler, where do you think the bullet is located?'"

"Did he really call you Doctor, Dr. Kessler?" a young woman said.

"Oh, yeah. McGill medical students were always addressed as 'Doctor' from Day One."

"That's cool."

"We thought so. Anyway, I told Dr. Penfield I thought the bullet was in the middle cranial *fossa* at the anterior tip of the right temporal lobe. So we had a problem.

"Dr. Cohen suggested we get a spinal tap. If there was blood in the fluid, then the bullet had entered the middle cranial *fossa* and they would have to open her skull. They did the spinal tap and it was positive for blood. So they proceeded to operate and removed the bullet. It had entered the left side of the girl's nose, leaving just a small scratch, passed through the top of the nasal cavity, entered the orbit, injured a vein which bled and caused the eyeball to bulge out The bullet then went out the back of the orbit and came to rest inside the cranial cavity.

"After the operation, Dr. Cohen asked me why I had ordered an X-ray even though it wasn't indicated by her history. I told him it was just dumb luck. That seemed to make him feel better. He wasn't dealing with a competitive boy genius or even an idiot savant. Just another green kid with a lot to learn. So he was free to allow my little blip to vanish from his radar screen. I doubt that either Dr. Penfield or Dr. Cohen retained any memory of my involvement in the case for more than a month or so. But I've never forgotten it."

"So what happened to the patient, Dr. Kessler?"

"Oh, yeah, the patient! The most important person in the story. That's always an excellent question. Well, Renata Heidersdorf had an uneventful recovery. Beyond that, I don't know."

"Did you start your surgical residency after graduating from McGill?

"No, I didn't. In those days, we had to take a 12-month rotating internship in medicine, surgery, pediatrics, obstetrics and emergency room care to become a general practitioner.

"After that, I decided to fulfill my two-year military obligation and get that out of the way. The U.S. wasn't at war with anybody at the time, but we still had the draft. I spent those years as an Army doctor in France. As an officer, I was making excellent money for the first time in my life and I can honestly say that those two years were some of the happiest I've ever had."

I made the final cut with my scissors and released the last adhesion in the cadaver's abdomen. Now that I had completed that boring, time-consuming task, I could start teaching and show my students some normal anatomy. I demonstrated the small bowel emptying into the large bowel and explained what the 'rosebud' showed us.

"It's the stoma of an isolated segment of ileum – a part of the small bowel. That tells us that we'll find a new urinary bladder. I'm sure the original bladder has been removed due to cancer. When you're dissecting in this man's pelvis, you'll be able to confirm that. Now we have to find the two ureters draining into this isolated loop of bowel. It's called an 'ileal bladder' by the way."

I showed them how to locate a ureter up near the kidney and trace it down to the ileal bladder. Apparently, the story of my medical training in the Dark Ages was more fascinating than my search for the isolated loop of small bowel, because a student asked me where I did my residency.

"After I got out of the Army, I did a four-year surgical residency in the District of Columbia at the Washington Hospital Center. But, wait! I've got it – the right ureter! So now I want all of you to take turns and reach inside and feel the right kidney. Don't all jump at once. Just feel it and notice that it's almost twice the normal size – and that you don't see any left ureters crossing over the mid-line. I think I know why."

I waited until all my students had felt the right kidney and then moved them to the other side of the cadaver's abdomen so that they could each palpate the left kidney. I then stepped back to watch them sticking their hands in the left upper quadrant of the dead man's abdomen, a little less gingerly now.

"Okay," I said, "we've now all found that the left kidney is very small, just as I suspected, and I'm sure it was non-functional because of some disease. To deal with that, the urologist who created this man's new bladder didn't bother to use the left ureters to drain the left kidney. Why didn't he?"

"Because the kidney wasn't working?"

"Right, that's pretty obvious. But, think about what's happening here. We don't know this guy's name or where he came from, but he's telling us a lot about himself – stuff we didn't know until we opened him up."

While I waited for all the students to compare the size of both kidneys, one of the young men asked if I had ever been in private practice. I told him I had a private practice in Ithaca, New York – but only for one year."

"I went to Cornell," he said. "I thought Ithaca was an okay town. Why did you leave?"

"Eighty per cent of my work was general practice. I felt I wouldn't be doing many of the major operations I'd been trained to do. So I came to New York City and got a full-time position at the Veterans Administration Hospital down the street. That was in 1964. We became affiliated with NYU in 1967. Another big reason I left Ithaca was that there was more opportunity to do research which I loved.

"Now," I said to the group, "if everyone has compared the two kidneys, let's think about what our friend here has taught you today. There's an old saying that we shouldn't judge a book by its cover. That's true for human beings, the living as well the dead. We shouldn't jump to conclusions. You didn't and I congratulate you on that.

"When you got your first look at our friend, you saw the 'rosebud' and you didn't know what it was. You didn't ignore that unexpected bit of information and start to make an incision. Instead, you asked someone with more experience for guidance. And that's something you should continue to do for the rest of your life in medicine. 'What is this thing?' you asked. Just simple curiosity led to what amounts to your first surgical consultation. That kept you from making a mistake, and it gave you a chance to see how to deal with the unexpected. You also learned something that most doctors 50 years ago knew nothing about."

"I guess you've seen a lot of changes in medicine," a young man said.

"You bet I have. Fifty years ago, we didn't have CT scans, MRIs, laparoscopic surgery, joint replacements and on and on. We practiced standard medicine with 15 or 20 drugs, three or four antibiotics, the usual narcotics for pain, plus aspirin and Tylenol for fevers. We had antihistamine and codeine medicine for colds, digitalis and nitroglycerine for the heart, tincture of belladonna and antacids for ulcers, and a dangerous mercurial diuretic for edema. And, of course, insulin for diabetes. For tranquilizers there was Thorazine and Compazine; several barbiturates for sleeping pills; and Novocain as a local anesthetic. Believe it or not, we thought we were hot shots in those days, but we didn't know *nuttin.*"

The students were too young to get my 'didn't know *nuttin'* reference, but they were beginning to chuckle as I took them down memory lane. That's always a good sign during the first month in the anatomy lab. They were starting to relax.

"Come to think of it," I said, "over the past 50 years, even the cadavers have changed. Back then, almost all the cadavers we studied were unclaimed bodies of indigent patients. Today, almost all of the cadavers have been donated by the deceased. It's a very noble way for people to dispose of their remains."

"Do you mean they're physically different?"

"In many ways, they are. As you've seen today, when you open up a body, you may find new heart valves, new coronary arteries, new hips and new knees. In many cadavers, the aorta has been replaced and new arteries have been grafted into the legs.

"We used to see a lot of gold fillings in the teeth, but dentists nowadays use different material. The man on the table was 88-years-old when he died. I'll bet he has some gold teeth. Let's take a look." The students froze. They stood wide-eyed and silent as I knew they would.

THE FIRST SESSION in a human anatomy lab is always a tense experience for young people. For most, it's the first time they actually confront the dead, face to face. The removal of the head wrappings is especially riveting. They are, after all, looking at the lifeless face of someone who was once as alive as they are now, someone's father or mother, perhaps. I've found that, from this point on, their relationship with the cadaver they study becomes personal. They wonder what kind of lives the cadavers had led and how they came to be here. Some give their cadavers names. And, after their final exam, some students return to the lab to say a prayer and thank their cadavers for their generosity.

But on this day, the young men and women weren't eager to have the hood and cloth wrappings removed from the head of the dead body, much less look at its face. It took some gentle persuasion to get them to watch me uncover the old man's head. They stood without flinching and stared at his light brown, leathery skin, his sunken cheeks, his lifeless eyes.

Death had taken the air out of him and his body had collapsed into itself. The blood, which had given his flesh, his veins and arteries and his vital organs their vibrancy and color, had been drained away by the embalmer. His eyes were sunken and his cheekbones prominent. His mouth was stretched open to reveal his teeth. Sure enough, a couple of them were gold. I didn't say I had told them so. I just let them look at the cadaver's face for a while before I replaced the wrappings.

"Now I want you to take a look at the body at the next table," I said. "We'll examine something we almost *never* saw 50 years ago. Take a look at that hole in the upper left quadrant of the woman's abdomen.

"That hole was made to allow passage of a tube into the stomach. The procedure's called a feeding gastrostomy and it's used to provide nourishment for patients who can't swallow but are still functional and neurologically intact. It's appropriate for patients with cancer of the throat or the esophagus.

"But, unfortunately, this procedure is now being applied to almost all patients who can't swallow, including those who've had massive strokes and have lost most, or all of their cognitive powers. Why do I say *unfortunately*?" I told the students to take a closer look.

"As you can see, this woman's left arm and left leg are atrophied. Note the severe contractures at her elbow and knee. That comes from lousy nursing care. This woman languished for a long time in a nursing home, I'll bet. She probably wasn't aware of very much.

"Fifty years ago, no one did gastrostomies in stroke patients like this poor lady. It wasn't considered humane to prolong the inevitable. When you open her head later on in the semester, you'll probably find that a large amount of the right side of her brain is gone."

By now, I could see that students from several other tables had come over to listen to my quiet tirade, so I continued: "You young people are all healthy now, but a serious auto accident tomorrow could render you brain dead. So I advise you to make out a Living Will now, specifying what you want and what you don't want to be done to you. That way you can avoid being trapped like this old lady or like that young woman in Florida."

"Are you referring to the Terri Schiavo case?"

"You bet I am. That young woman and her family were in a terrible situation. The meddling of a lot of self-serving politicians only made it worse. I have a living will that specifically forbids the use of a feeding tube, IVs, transfusions, dialysis, respirator and any other 'extraordinary' tools or procedures.

"If I'm so neurologically compromised that I can't make a decision for myself, I don't want to languish in a nursing home getting bedsores and joint contractures, pissing my pants, soiling the sheets, and being unable to communicate my emotional agony. I want to let go and depart without some eager doctor extending my terminal state.

"Some lawyers call it 'TTPG – Trying to Play God.' Back in the 1930s, Pope Pius XII made it quite clear in one of his encyclicals that it wasn't the duty of the medical profession to prolong the misery of a terminal patient, but merely to make the person as calm and comfortable as possible.

"The treatment this poor woman got didn't do her any good and probably did a lot of financial harm to her family – if she had one. It costs $60,000 a year to be in a nursing home and once Medicare runs out, the family picks up the tab. So, make out a living will. That's what this old lady is telling you."

I joined some other students at the far end of the lab who were also encountering some problem with their cadaver and needed help. "We've been exploring the abdomen and we've found this structure coming out through the abdominal wall. What is it?"

It was another 'rosebud'– this time in the left lower quadrant. They had come across a colostomy or a segment of large bowel.

"The stool comes out through that 'rosebud' into a bag," I told them. "This patient either had a serious infection or cancer in the lower part of the colon or rectum. When you dissect the pelvis, you'll be able to see what's missing."

"That must be hard to live with," a student remarked.

"Not necessarily. A colostomy can be trained to evacuate each morning with an enema. As a matter of fact, Winston Churchill had one of these for 45 years."

"Is that going to be on the final exam, Doctor?"

"Probably not," I said. "If I decide otherwise, I'll put Churchill's bag in a True or False section."

ANOTHER REWARDING DAY. Once again, I realized why I continued to teach instead of retiring completely. Staying in contact with students renewed my hope in the future. But over the years, I had observed the medical school's enrollment changing as the practice of medicine became more onerous. A former colleague of mine, who had been called out of retirement to help interview applicants for admission to medical school, told me that very few of the young men and women who had applied were the children of American doctors.

I haven't come across any statistics to suggest that's a national trend, but discouraging your child from following in your professional footsteps might be a symptom of something that's been going wrong. As I said before, the practice of medicine in the United States *used* to be fun.

When I started out the first thing we'd ask a patient was, "What seems to be wrong?" Nowadays, the first question for patients has to do with what, if any, medical insurance they have.

THE DEADLY RED SPOT

O NCE EACH SEMESTER, I give a lecture on the anatomy of the human butt. Call it what you will – the rump, Keister, can, rear end, derriere or the ass – it's an important topic for my first-year medical students. I use slides and blackboard drawings to illustrate my discussion of the various bones, ligaments, nerves, blood vessels and muscles located in the buttocks. One of my slides, made from a diagram in *Grant's Atlas of Anatomy*, beautifully depicts the largest muscle in the human body, the gluteus maximus, which forms the bulk of the butt.

This lecture, while important, runs the risk of being tedious and boring for medical students because it contains a lot of mundane anatomical trivia that has little clinical significance. Probably, the only salient point for doctors-to-be is where to put a needle when injecting medication into a patient's backside. To help my students remember, I tell them about an experience I had when I was a first-year medical student myself. I was ill with a high fever and sore throat.

The university sent a young internist to my boarding house to examine me. That was back in the age of dinosaurs when doctors still made house calls. The young doctor determined that I had a strep-throat infection and gave me a shot of Penicillin – right in the middle of my buttocks! A horrible pain sped from my butt down to my foot and I screamed – loudly!

"What happened?" gasped the young doctor.

I rolled over and growled. "You put the goddam needle through my damn sciatic nerve!"

"I couldn't have!"

"Well, you did! Hand me that anatomy text over there on my desk. I'll *show* you what you did!"

I opened the anatomy book to the gluteal region section and showed him the sciatic nerve. "Right there! It's the biggest nerve in the body, for crying out loud!" I proclaimed this with the authority of one who had just reviewed the human butt the week before. And then I showed him the diagram of the entire rear end.

"All buttocks are divided into four parts," I growled. "The next time you stick a needle into somebody's ass, make sure you stick it in the upper outer quadrant!" At which point, I glare at my students. "And that goes for you people, too!"

That always gets a big laugh. Former students have told me that the story of the needle plunged into Dr. Kessler's Keister stuck in their memory for 20 years or more. At any rate, once my current students become fully awake and stop laughing, I tell them about another personal experience I had some years before.

I'D GONE TO FLORIDA to visit my Dad. He'd had a mini-stroke and was hospitalized in the town of Spring Hill on the Gulf Coast north of Tampa. Dad had been in a coma for several days, so there was really nothing I could do for him except sit by his bed with my childhood memories and be there with him.

Dad had been the principal of the school I went to in Theresa, a small town in Upstate New York, about an hour's drive from the St. Lawrence River. Dad made sure I got a good education, but no special privileges. The winters were long and cold up there and money was scarce when I was a kid. I remembered sitting at the crossroads in January selling Sunday newspapers to people hurrying home from church – and wishing I lived someplace warm. Now here I was in hot and humid Florida. Thank goodness for the air conditioning!

A nurse entered the room to change the bed linen and give Dad his daily back care. When she turned him on his side, I noticed a red spot the size of a dime on his buttocks over the sacrum.

"Do you see that red spot over my Dad's tailbone?" I asked the nurse. "Do you know what it means?"

"Yes, I do."

"We won't be seeing that red spot tomorrow, will we, Nurse?"

"No, we won't," she said. "I'll take care of it." And, sure enough, the next day the red spot was gone.

"THAT SAVED MY DAD a lot of grief," I tell my students. "He recovered from his stroke uneventfully and he lived another three years before an aortic aneurysm ruptured. But let me show you what my Dad avoided because that nurse and I noticed that little red spot and did something about it."

That's when I show them slides of horrendous pressure sores and begin my explanation. "A decubitus ulcer or bedsore," I tell them, "is actually a pressure sore that develops from prolonged pressure on the skin that covers bone. This prolonged pressure interrupts the blood supply to the structures superficial to bony prominences and that results in tissue breakdown. The areas most vulnerable are the back of the head, the base of the spine, the side of the hips, the bones we sit on and the heels.

"Constant pressure for no more than two hours is sufficient to cause tissue breakdown. The patients who are most vulnerable are the malnourished, the immobilized and those who are unable to feel the discomfort of constant pressure – paraplegics, people in comas, people who have been over-dosed with drugs. Healthy people don't get bedsores during sleep because they toss and turn unconsciously in response to the uncomfortable stimulus of remaining in one position too long.

"Remember," I tell them, "the red spot is the first indication of a pressure sore on the skin. If the patient is allowed to remain in that position, the skin will soon break down and become an ulcer. If the pressure continues, the ulcer gets bigger, deeper and infected. Eventually it will involve muscle and bone. Sometimes the infection can be so severe as to cause death."

Now, with the students completely focused and sitting straight up in their chairs, I stress that the best treatment for a bedsore is prevention. "And you prevent a bedsore by the simple act of turning the patient at least every two hours," I tell them. "There are special mattresses, beds and cushions that have been devised to aid in prevention and treatment. But these ancillary measures should never replace the requirement of turning a patient frequently when they cannot do it themselves.

"Families who are taking care of aging and debilitated bedridden relatives at home often find it almost impossible to turn the patient every two hours. Under these circumstances, the development of bedsores is unfortunate, but understandable. After all, most families don't have the financial resources to hire around-the-clock nurses. But hospital-acquired bedsores, on the other hand, are almost always the result of inadequate nursing care and are a common cause of litigation."

ON THIS DAY, LITIGATION was very much on my mind. The jury was still out on a malpractice case in which I had testified as an expert witness for the plaintiff and I couldn't help wondering about the final outcome. I saw a hand go up and that got my mind back to the business at hand.

"Dr. Kessler, you talked about paraplegics being vulnerable to pressure sores. I didn't understand why. They can shift around in their wheelchairs, can't they?"

"Well, yes, many can. But consider this: you've been sitting here in a chair listening to my lecture which you have undoubtedly found fascinating. Even so, you've been shifting from one side of your buttocks to the other. Why? Not because you're bored, I'm sure, but because you've found it uncomfortable to remain in the same position for very long.

"But a paraplegic can't feel the discomfort because the pain pathways in the spinal cord have been interrupted by the back injury. So the paraplegic may stay in one position so long that the skin begins to break down. These patients have been advised to shift their weight in their wheelchair every half hour or so. If they forget, they may develop a pressure sore."

"Do they have to be hospitalized for treatment of these skin breakdowns?"

"I think most of them should be hospitalized, especially if they live alone. After all, most of these bedsores are on the buttocks. So the patient may have difficulty taking care of an ulcer that is out of sight. I know of one case where a middle-aged paraplegic who lived alone developed a one-inch pressure sore on her buttocks shortly after being discharged from the hospital after undergoing a hysterectomy. Her doctor opted to treat her sore on an outpatient basis with debridement and primary suturing.

"The suture line broke down and over the next three years she was treated by visiting nurses, occasional brief hospitalization for surgery, followed by premature discharge and visiting nurses *ad infinitum*. She eventually developed three pressure sores. The largest measured 10 by 16 centimeters and was nine centimeters deep, thus invading muscle and bone. When you think about it, it would have cost a lot less money if they had treated her properly when the ulcer was small, clean and superficial."

"When we become doctors," a young woman asked, "how often can we expect to see bedsores as bad as the ones you showed us on the slides?"

I looked at her and was suddenly struck by the thought that my students seemed to be getting younger every year. I shook my head. "Bedsores are very common and the incidence of bedsores seems to be increasing."

"Why is that?" she asked.

"Well, most hospitals have had to cut the number of nurses they employ. Each nurse has an increased workload and so nurses can't devote as much time to each patient as they did 20 years ago."

"But why do hospitals have to cut their nursing staffs?"

"The short answer is money," I said. "There are other reasons, of course. But, right now, let's stick to medicine, not politics. If you want my opinions, see me after the lecture. Are there any other questions about bedsores?"

"Which kinds of hospitals are most likely to have problems with bedsores?" a young man asked.

"Hospitals with poor supervision. But the most dreadful bedsore cases I've seen have involved people transferred from nursing homes to general hospitals for treatment."

"Do they get bedsores at your VA Hospital?"

"Rarely. It's been many years since I've seen a bedsore develop at the Manhattan VA Hospital. The ones we treat result from poor care in nursing homes."

"Why is that?"

"The incidence of bedsores in any institution largely depends on the motivation and the authority of its Director of Nursing. The best one I've ever known is down the street at the VA Hospital. We have a lot of old, debilitated veterans and if there's the beginning of a bedsore – a red spot – the shit really hits the fan. Furthermore, no patient is ever sent home with a red spot, let alone an existing bedsore."

"My Grandmother was sent home with a bedsore that developed in a hospital," said a student who seldom spoke up in class.

"Did it heal at home?"

"No, it didn't," he answered. "It got worse."

"I have heard that story many times before," I said. "Not that it's any consolation for you. Not too long ago, a law firm asked me to review the chart of an elderly bedridden nurse who had developed a decubitus ulcer in the hospital. She was discharged and sent home with an ulcer on her buttocks that was the size of a quarter. Her family wasn't equipped to deal with it, especially since she was incontinent and could no longer control her bladder or bowel functions.

"Ten days later, she had to be re-admitted to the hospital because the ulcer had grown to the size of a silver dollar and it was because of necrotic tissue – dead tissue. The woman had to stay hospitalized for six weeks and she underwent major plastic surgery. It would have been better and cheaper for her if she hadn't been sent home too soon. If she'd stayed in the hospital the first time, aggressive nursing care could have healed the ulcer in just a few days."

"Are there many hospitals like that?"

"There shouldn't be any, but there are some," I said. "There's one stinking institution here in the New York metropolitan area that's been sued so many times that it ought to be shut down. I know of one elderly lady who was admitted to that hospital following a stroke. Two and one half weeks later, she was transferred to a nursing home with 17 – yes, 17! – bedsores. When she arrived, the nursing home administrator took photographs to document the woman's sorry condition – to cover his own ass from a lawsuit, of course. I wish I had those photos to show you. You wouldn't believe how bad nursing care can get in some hospitals and nursing homes."

"WHEN YOU BECOME DOCTORS," I tell my first-year medical students, "you will be caring for bedridden patients. Each day, when you make your rounds, it will be your duty to turn the patient and look for that little red spot or – God forbid! – an ulcer. And whenever you find evidence of a pressure sore developing, it will be your duty to go to the nurse in charge and rant and rave, stamp your feet, curse and yell and inform the nurses to get off their own derrieres and do their jobs properly.

"It's much easier and cheaper to prevent bedsores than to treat them. Once they develop into big, deep, infected wounds, hospitalization is lengthy and the major plastic surgery required is expensive. As I said: bedsores can get so bad they can kill people! That's a fact! Always remember that – and always remember to check your patients to make sure they don't have a little red spot anywhere on their backsides."

I make a show of gathering up my slides and notes. "Oh, yeah," I say. "There's one more thing to remember. If you have to give your patient a shot in the butt, make sure you stick the needle in the upper outer quadrant. That's it for today." They usually leave laughing – most of them. But a few students always hang around to ask questions.

"Dr. Kessler, about the reduction of nursing staffs being one cause of the increase of bedsores? You said the short answer was money. What's the long answer?"

"You're a very persistent young lady, aren't you? Well, that's good. But before I answer, I want to make something clear. What I'm going to say is my own opinion. It's based on my own experience and observation over a long career. And I know there are plenty of doctors and politicians and pundits who won't agree with me. I'm speaking for myself now, not for the school. Got it?"

"I understand," she said. "This is un-official."

"That's correct. Strictly my own opinion. Now let me say that I believe the incidence of bedsores seems to be increasing, along with some other preventable things, because in today's medical environment the emphasis seems to be on cost-effectiveness and profit for shareholders and insurance companies."

"So what do you think can be done about it?"

"Frankly, I think we need a national health care system funded by the tax payer. But as long as the voters keep electing government officials who promise to cut taxes and cut spending, there will never be adequate funds for important social needs."

"That sounds like socialized medicine," said a young man.

"Yes, it is," I said with a smile. "At least, that's what some people call it. But we have Social Security and Medicare and Medicaid without which a lot of senior citizens couldn't survive. And let's not forget an old and well-established organization that provides socialized medicine to the men and women who served our country in the armed forces. The Veterans Administration provides excellent health care and does it very economically."

I looked at my watch. "I'd like to hang around and convert all of you to my way of thinking, but the VA requires my presence at the hospital just about now. Thank goodness, it's not that far away."

I WAS EAGER TO FIND OUT the result of the trial I'd testified at three days before over in Queens. It had been a case of an obese elderly woman who had developed a horrendous bedsore. She'd become critically ill and bed-ridden following her surgery for gangrenous bowel in a strangulated, umbilical hernia. I had testified that the huge bedsore, which almost killed the patient from infection, was preventable with proper nursing care.

During my testimony, the judge hearing the case demonstrated his bias by reading my testimony in a similar case several years before in which I'd testified for another plaintiff. The judge was helping the defense lawyers in their effort to find a contradiction with which to impeach me. The judge seemed disappointed when he couldn't find one. I wasn't too shocked. I'd encountered judges before who did not seem to use good judgment, but this one took the prize. At one point, when I testified that I had treated heart attacks when I was medical director of an emergency room, the judge (with the jury present) interjected: "That's nothing. Even a boy scout can handle an emergency."

Later in the trial, when I gave an answer to a question that had been put to me, the judge said – in front of the jury – that he would have allowed my answer if I had never testified before. But since I was an experienced witness, he would not allow the jury to consider my answer. When I left the witness stand, I whispered to the plaintiff's attorney, "Is he always like that?"

"Don't worry about it. You did fine. The judge is a disgrace. Everyone knows he's an asshole. Is that a medical term, Doctor?"

"Actually, in this case, it is," I said *sotto voce.* "And you used it correctly."

When I finished my dash from the medical school to the hospital, I found a message in my box from the lawyer. The verdict was in and the jury had awarded the woman $250,000. The members of the jury might not have been experts on human anatomy, but apparently they knew enough zoology to recognize a jackass when they heard one.

5

MY WAR AGAINST THE CLAP

━━━━

I WAS EARLY FOR MY 10 a.m. Anatomy class. The subject would be abdominal pain, but I was thinking about gonorrhea. I was going to present three cases to my first-year medical students and one of them involved a young woman who had contracted that venereal disease by not practicing safe sex. Her case would give me an excellent opportunity to introduce the students to the subject of spreading peritonitis as well as testing their knowledge of female pelvic anatomy. I wanted to get to the anatomy lab early so that I'd have plenty of time to check the female cadavers and select one that still had its pelvic organs intact.

As I walked up First Avenue from the VA Hospital to the NYU Medical School, I thought back to the numerous cases of Pelvic Inflammatory Disease (PID) I had treated during my residency in Washington, D.C. Most of those cases had been caused by gonorrhea and some of those cases had been so severe that they required surgery – even hysterectomy. When it comes to gonorrhea, women have a much tougher time of it than men.

In medical school, I had learned about the diagnosis and treatment of gonococcal urethritis in the male and had observed several cases that were easily treated with a single shot – 300,000 units of penicillin. But most of my experience with the disease came after my internship when I began my obligatory two years of service in the U.S. Army Medical Corps.

IN AUGUST OF 1957, I was stationed at an Army base in Rochefort, France, an area rich in history. Rochefort had been a French naval base for centuries. From here, the explorer Samuel de Champlain had sailed to explore the New World. Most of Rochefort's historic buildings had been demolished by the retreating Germans in the summer of 1944. The ancient buildings had been replaced by G.I. structures and metal Quonset huts. The base medical dispensary, which serviced about 1,500 troops and their families, was located next to Champlain's abandoned boat basin. The dispensary had three doctors, two dentists, 15 to 20 corpsmen and a cheerful warrant officer named Mr. Roberts who took care of the administrative paper work most doctors detest.

We had a busy, albeit routine, general practice. But Monday and Tuesday were our "gonorrhea days." A young soldier – and often more than one – would report for sick call complaining of burning on urination and yellow pus dripping from his penis. It took just a few minutes for Big Mac, our lab technician, to report that the soldier's distress was due to a gram-negative intracellular diplococcus. Or, as Big Mac would say, "The guy's got the clap, Sir."

It didn't take me long to realize that too many of our soldiers were getting infected in Rochefort's red-light district, the neighborhood known as "South-40." Rochefort's South-40 was unique. The Army usually designates red light districts as "Off Limits" to military personnel. Not so, South-40. For some reasons I never understood, the Army had declared Rochefort's South-40 "On Limits" in 1944 and it remained so, at least during my tour of duty.

It was definitely a public health problem. To my knowledge, South-40 was the only red light district in Western Europe where an American serviceman could go without fear of being harassed by the military police. That became common knowledge at all the other American bases in Europe and Rochefort soon became a magnet for servicemen on leave looking for a town where they could have some "fun" without getting arrested by the MPs.

As a doctor, I couldn't ignore what was going on in South-40 and I began putting two and two together. Rochefort's red light district, I finally concluded, was probably spreading venereal disease all over Europe. South-40 had to be closed down, I decided, or be cleaned up. So I began working my way up the Army's chain of command. I went first to my immediate superior, the CO of the base infirmary. He was a physician with the rank of captain in the Army Medical Corps. I asked him if he knew who the VD Control Officer on our base might be.

"I have no idea," he said. "Why are you asking?"

"South-40 is a cesspool of gonorrhea and we need to do something about it. The women need to be examined and tested for venereal diseases and treated."

The captain gave me a stricken look. "Look, Dick," he said, "I've got my hands full with this dispensary and, besides, I'm a Catholic, you know? I really don't want to get mixed up with the local whores."

"Then do I have your permission to go see the Colonel about this?"

"Oh, sure, Dick!" he said. "Please! Be my guest!"

So I went to see the commanding officer of the base, Colonel Dann. Besides being in charge of everything and everybody, the CO was the tallest man in camp. He stood six-feet-six-inches, which was as tall as you were allowed to be in the Army. He had made his mark in amphibious warfare during the Inchon landings in Korea.

Colonel Dann was a "mustang," one of those Army men who had come up through the ranks to become an officer. When I arrived in Rochefort, he was a capable, confident lieutenant colonel with an enlisted man's vocabulary. He never failed to greet those of us in the Medical Corps with that old Bugs Bunny line.

"Hey! What's up Doc?" he said as he casually returned my regulation salute.

"Sir, could you tell me who the VD control officer is here?"

"The Post Chaplain."

"You've got to be kidding!"

"I know it sounds ridiculous, Doc, but nobody else wants the fucking job. No pun intended."

"May I ask what the chaplain does to control VD?"

Colonel Dann leaned back in his chair, stretched out his arms, and yawned. "Well, Doc," he said, "the chaplain gives the boys a sermon every once in a while. He tells them they shouldn't do nasty things when they're on leave. Then he makes them look at that damn movie that shows what can happen to a soldier's dick if he catches a venereal disease. Actually, it's a pretty gruesome film. One guy's pecker spouts like a sprinkling can when he takes a piss. It's enough to make a GI swear off sex for a least a week. So, what's your problem, Doc?"

"We're seeing a lot of gonorrhea coming out of South-40."

"That doesn't surprise me, Doc, but I'd hate to close down the South-40 cat-houses. I like to know where my troops are when they're not here on the base."

"I don't want to shut them down either, Colonel. The girls would just start working the streets and that would make things even worse. We'd lose control completely."

"So what have you got in mind?"

"First off, I'd like to be made VD Control Officer"

"You bet, Doc! You've got it! Best news I've had all week!" He wrote on the yellow pad on his desk. "I'm reminding myself to let the chaplain know that he's off the hook. He hates showing that damn movie."

"Please don't do that, Sir," I said. "I think the chaplain should keep on giving his sex talks to the men and showing them his movie. I don't know how much good it does, probably not much, but it can't hurt."

"Yeah, maybe you're right. So what is it that *you* want to do, Doc? You've got some kind of plan in mind?"

"What I'd like to do, Colonel, is shut down South-40 for two weeks. During that two-week period, we'll give each prostitute a shot of long-acting penicillin. When the two weeks are up, South-40 can go back to business as usual. But from then on, the girls will get a shot of penicillin once every month. That should clean up the mess and keep our soldiers healthy and stop the spread of the clap to other bases in Europe."

Colonel Dann sat frowning for a few moments and then made some more notes on his yellow pad. "You know, Doc, I think General

MacArthur did something like that in Japan. He got pretty good results, I seem to recall. So, what the Hell! If it was a good enough for Macarthur, it's good enough for me. Do you know Red, our interpreter?"

"Not really, Sir," I said. "He's an Italian, isn't he?"

"Yeah, our guys captured him in North Africa during the war. Probably couldn't miss him with that shock of red hair. Anyhow, it turned out he was fluent in seven languages, so the Army started using him as a civilian interpreter. And now I've got him. I'll get Red to set up a meeting with the town madams so you can tell them what we want to do. Just between you and me, Doc, I can't prove it but I think Red's been moonlighting – pimping for any whores who happen to be passing through Rochefort."

"Sounds like setting up this meeting will be right up his alley, Sir. No pun intended."

"I guess you could say that. Doc. Red speaks their language, in more ways than one."

Red was a fast worker. Before the week was out, he had me back in the CO's office sitting with three formidable Frenchwomen of uncertain ages who had put on their best frocks and their best manners for this formal occasion. Colonel Dann solemnly greeted the women, thanked them for accepting our invitation and swiftly departed "with regret" to attend to some pressing military matters. That left me alone to explain, through Red, the Army's proposal for putting the women out of business for a full two weeks.

Sitting ramrod straight, the madams listened in silence. I could see that they were upset. When I had stopped speaking in English and Red had finished translating my English into French, the women exchanged glances. Without a single spoken word, they arrived at an agreement and chose a spokesperson, Madame Mickey – or *Mee-KEY,* as she pronounced it. (I learned later that Madame Mickey's real name was Gillette Scaramouche. She was an intelligent, experienced woman who began her professional career as a teenage prostitute when Kaiser Wilhelm's troops marched into France in the First World War.)

Madame Mickey spoke and Red interpreted her statement. "The good women of Rochefort," he said, "thank you for your courtesy and hospitality and wish you to know that it is their belief that The Boss would not be pleased to have his businesses shut down for two weeks."

"The Boss?" I said to Red. "Who the hell is this Boss?"

"Let us say that he is an important man in the community," Red replied with a shrug. "I'm told that he is a man of great influence. But, if you will pardon me, Doc, I believe the less you know about The Boss, the better. However, there is good news. The ladies propose that another meeting should take place in town, this time with The Boss in attendance. They hope their proposal meets with your approval."

"Tell the ladies I would be pleased to attend such a meeting. And as soon as possible. Tell them I'd like to include the local French doctor who looks after the health of the young women in their employ, since he would be the one to administer the penicillin shots to the . . . the . . ." My mind had gone blank.

"The whores," said Red. "Don't worry, Doc. I'll use a proper French word. An interpreter must be a diplomat as well as a translator."

So the meeting, like most business meetings, concluded with a general agreement to have another meeting. "Nice going, Doc," Red said *sotto voce*. "You've made a good impression and moved your case forward. I'll see the ladies to their vehicle."

Before leaving, Madame Mickey shook my hand and thanked me for the Army's hospitality – in English. "And please, Dr. Kessler, express my thanks to your Colonel Dann. He is a handsome, charming man and he has been a good neighbor. Please tell him to come by sometime to pay me a visit and I shall assure him a good fuck."

"I shall, Madame," I said with a slight bow. "I'll tell the Colonel when he returns. I can hardly wait to do so."

My next meeting with the madams of Rochefort was scheduled for the following week at a hotel owned by The Boss. I wanted to impress The Boss and show him who was in charge. So I decked myself out in my dress blue uniform hoping to look more like a military officer than a doctor. But the callow young man looking back from my mirror looked like someone from the Civil War – a tall, skinny, awkward Union Army recruit. I decided that charm and logic would have to be my weapons, not intimidation.

Red disagreed. He gave me a pep talk as we walked to the meeting. "Don't forget that you are dealing with Europeans, Doc – and French ones, at that. They don't understand how things are done in America. If you're polite and friendly, they'll take it as a sign of weakness. So don't treat them as equals. Let them know that you speak for the whole damn American Army and that they damn well better pay attention. Don't be a good guy. Be stern and forceful. And don't let The Boss scare you. But, for my sake, please try not to piss him off."

I took a deep breath, squared my shoulders, and advanced on the hotel. Once inside, Red and I were ushered down a corridor to a dramatically lit parlor with dark walls, overstuffed chairs and fringed table lamps. It seemed as if I had stumbled onto the set of a *film noir* melodrama. Red did his best to bolster my image by introducing me to the seven madams and the local doctor as "*Capitaine* Kessler."

Red did *not* introduce me to the heavy set, square-jawed man sitting in the shadows with his back to the corner of the room. This was The Boss – a European mobster straight from Central Casting. He did not look up when I entered the room and never once during the meeting did he look me straight in the eye. His feigned indifference, I decided, was a ploy to make himself more important and more menacing than he possibly could be – probably just a pimp trying to pass himself off as a tough guy. Well, I would show him what tough was.

Fortunately, it was not until weeks later that I learned that the man in the dark corner controlled all the gambling, prostitution and narcotic rackets in that region of France. He owned hundreds of acres of poppy fields. And there were rumors that gangsters who tried to muscle in on The Boss's territory wound up floating down the Charente River to the sea.

Unburdened by any of this intelligence, I stood tall and confidently spoke my piece. "South-40 is a dirty, rotten cesspool!" I slapped the palm of my hand on a table, hard. "South-40 is rampant with the clap and it's got to stop! If you do not do what I say, the American Army will place South-40 off limits. Off Limits! Then you will have only French sailors and civilians for clients! But no American soldiers! Not one! And this district will be patrolled by American military police! All this will be bad for your business because, I understand, the French sailor pays only one third of what the American soldier pays."

I waited until Red translated what I had said into French. "All this can be avoided," I continued, "but only if you agree to do what I say. I have a proposal to make and I want you to hear me out and consider it carefully."

I was addressing my remarks to the madams, never speaking directly to The Boss. I watched Madame Mickey glance in his direction and, from the corner of my eye, saw him nod his head ever so slightly. So I went on to explain my plan for shutting down South-40 for two weeks, giving the prostitutes an initial shot of penicillin and, after business resumed, giving each one additional shots every month. "In this way," I explained, "the germ that causes the clap will be eradicated. And that will be better for everyone concerned. I hope we can all agree to this plan of attack."

This time, after Red finished translating, all of the madams looked to the dark corner for guidance and, once again, the man in the shadows nodded his approval. But the French doctor had a question. "Who will give these shots?" said Red, translating.

"Tell him that he will," I said.

The doctor had more questions. "Suppose someone is allergic to penicillin?" he asked in French.

"They can not ever work in South-40."

"Suppose someone has an anaphylactic reaction to penicillin?"

"*C'est la guerre*," I replied. "If they can't get a shot, they can't work in South-40."

The French doctor threw up his hands "This long-acting penicillin causes pain in the buttocks for two or three days. As you know, these women make their living on their buttocks. That could be a problem."

I shook off his appeal. "Once the word is out that Rochefort has a clean, safe operation here, the houses will be so busy that they'll be able to afford giving their women some extra days off. And let me add that any new girls who come to town will be obliged to get a shot of penicillin and wait two weeks before beginning work."

The man in the corner stood up and began to move toward the door, leaving no doubt that the meeting was over. As The Boss passed in front of me, he honored me with a curt nod of his head. I gave him one back. The Boss and I had reached an agreement without a single word passing between us.

The prophylactic plan went into effect almost immediately. And, for the next 18 months, our base dispensary did not see a single case of VD come out of South-40. From time to time, some of our soldiers did show up with gonorrhea or syphilis or chancroid. But they had picked up those diseases in places like Place Pigale, Piccadilly or – in one case – Hamburg, West Germany.

THE FRENCH NAVY had a hospital in the Rochefort area and I had become quite friendly with its chief of staff, a French naval officer who was a physician and spoke fluent English. He sometimes asked me to accompany him on rounds and showed me many fascinating cases in his wards, including one I had never seen before: scrofula. It's a disease that develops from drinking un-pasteurized milk and it leads to tuberculosis in the neck.

"Is it not amazing," the French doctor said, "how so many people in the land of Louis Pasteur still drink the raw milk?" When I visited him a few weeks after the American prophylactic plan became operational in Rochefort, he told me that his hospital was seeing significantly fewer cases of VD among the French sailors. "Congratulations, *Mon Ami!* Your program is working!"

Nevertheless, my campaign to stamp out sexual disease and pestilence in South-40 almost came to a halt one year after it began. It had been a good year. I had become CO of the base infirmary and had moved to a small villa out beyond Rochefort on the Atlantic shore. I was hosting a dinner one quiet Sunday afternoon when one of Madame Mickey's girls came knocking at my kitchen door. "Madame apologizes for bothering you on a Sunday," she said, "but Madame says it's very important."

I followed her down the walk to the huge Cadillac parked in front of my house where Madame Mickey, ensconced in the back seat, gave me the bad news. "They are going to close South-40," she said. "Some new generals up in Orleans, they are making South-40 off limits."

"I haven't heard anything about that, Mickey. Are you sure? How do you know?"

"I have ways of knowing many things. I knew always what the Germans were doing and I know now what you Americans are doing. You will learn about this tomorrow, officially."

That Monday morning, I arrived at Colonel Dann's office at 8:00 a.m. – sharp.

"What's up, Doc?" he asked. "As if I couldn't guess. You've heard. How'd you find out so soon? I just opened the damn orders five minutes ago!"

"Madame Mickey told me yesterday. She was so upset that she drove out to my place to give me the news."

"How the hell did she know yesterday? What kind of security do we have around here anyway? It's a damn wonder we ever won a war."

"Who are these new generals?"

"Some more ring-knockers, I suppose. Tight-ass West Pointers. They don't want to have it on their record that they're condoning immoral behavior. But stupidity is okay, I guess. Maybe I can get the chaplain to show them his VD movie." Colonel Dann smacked his fist in the palm of his left hand. "When I calm down, I'll call Orleans and tell them how General Douglas MacArthur's VD prevention program is working great right here in Rochefort, just like it did in Japan. Isn't that what the local newspapermen call it? The MacArthur Plan?"

"Not to my knowledge, Colonel."

"Well, they do now, Doc. At least, that's what I'll tell them up in Orleans." He gave me a wave of the hand. "Go back to work, Doc. I'll handle this. Don't you worry."

He did handle it, but he never told me how. At any rate, Orleans HQ rescinded the "Off Limits" order and VD in Rochefort remained virtually eradicated – at least on our base. Unfortunately, some French people in the town still got sick because they didn't practice what is known today as "safe sex." But, then, some people in the town still got sick from drinking raw milk.

6

THE CLAP GOES MARCHING ON

![divider]

ALL THAT WAS YESTERDAY. I was no longer the idealistic young American Army officer known throughout the red-light district of Rochefort, France, as *"Le Capitaine"* – the man who brought a dose of sanity and penicillin to South-40, a man so respected that no one would allow him to pay for a drink or a meal. Four decades had passed and on this morning I was just a professor standing in the NYU anatomy lab waiting for my idealistic young students to join me and my cadavers to discuss, among other things, "the clap." I reminded myself that this was a medical school, not the Army, and the ten young students entering the lab were not soldiers. Here, among the dead, we call organs and diseases by their proper names – most of the time.

The students signed the attendance sheet and gathered around the cadaver I had selected: a female with pelvic organs intact. On the adjacent table, I had placed the lower half of a female cadaver that had been bisected down the middle. That specimen would be useful for testing their knowledge of the blood vessels and nerves in the pelvis.

"The case I want to discuss with you," I began, "concerns a very common condition that most of you will see in your clinical practice, especially if you see patients in the ER. The patient is a young female in her early twenties. She enters the ER complaining of severe abdominal pain. She walks stooped over and each step escalates the pain. Each step makes it worse. Her pain started five days ago and has gradually worsened. She now has a fever of 102, a rapid pulse and her white blood count is elevated. It's obvious she has an infection in her abdominal cavity. This is called peritonitis and there are many conditions that can cause it."

I placed my hands on the left lower quadrant of the cadaver's abdomen and asked a student, "What organs are located in this region that might become infected and cause peritonitis?"

"The large bowel," he answered.

"Can you be more specific?"

"The sigmoid colon."

"That's correct. An infection in the sigmoid colon is usually caused by diverticulae – sacs in the bowel – that have become infected. This is referred to as diverticulitis. The pain begins in the left lower quadrant. If the infection gets worse, the pain will spread to other areas of the abdomen. What organs in the left upper quadrant might become infected and cause pain in that region?" I asked a young woman.

"The spleen," she answered without hesitation.

"Anything else?"

"Maybe, the pancreas?"

"That's right. Absolutely. We call that pancreatitis. What else?"

"I don't know," she admitted.

"Anyone?" I asked.

"The stomach?" several students replied.

"Correct. Infection in the stomach is called gastritis. What about the right upper quadrant?"

"The liver?"

"Sure," I said. "And that's called hepatitis."

"The gall bladder," said the next student.

"Yes, an infection in the gall bladder is a very common condition called cholecystitis. Now, what about the right lower quadrant?"

"The large bowel."

"OK. What else?"

"How about the appendix?"

"Yes, indeed. An infection in the appendix, as you know, is called appendicitis. The pain begins in the right lower quadrant. As the infection gets worse, it spreads to other areas of the abdomen. What else?"

"A cyst on the ovary," a student suggested.

"Right. That can cause lower abdominal pain if the cyst ruptures. But that is not an infection."

A young man who seldom spoke in class said, "What about an ectopic pregnancy?"

"That's very good! It can cause severe pain in the lower abdomen. But where did a first-year medical student hear about ectopic pregnancy?"

"My cousin had it happen to her."

"Well, then, perhaps you can tell the other students what that is."

"It's a pregnancy in the fallopian tube that ruptures and bleeds."

"He's absolutely correct," I told the other students. "And what else can cause severe pain in the lower quadrants?" I asked a young woman.

"An infection in the tubes," she replied.

"Absolutely. That's called salpingitis. And salpingitis plays a part in the case we're talking about today. But we'll get back to that later. Right now, on this bisected specimen, please show me the cervix and cervical canal."

She did and I said to the group gathered around the table, "You can see where an infection in the cervix can spread upwards into the uterine cavity." I asked the next student to show me the uterine cavity and the uterus. He pointed them out and I asked him, "What's the blood supply to the uterus?"

"The uterine artery and the ovarian artery," he answered and showed me where they were. And so it went around the table with the students pointing out the broad ligament, the cardinal ligament, the round ligament, the vagina and posterior fornix, the sacro-uterine ligament, and the ovary. I kept moving them along with questions and commands: What is the blood supply to the ovary? Show me the ligament of the ovary. Show me the ovarian artery. Show me the mesovarium. Show me the meso-salpinx.

"Okay," I said to them finally. "Good job. You know your stuff. So, let's return to our case study. We need to talk about the pelvic examination. During a vaginal examination of a PID patient, a slight movement of the cervix from one side to the other causes severe abdominal pain. Can anyone tell me why that is?"

After a long pause without an answer in sight, I explained that in patients with PID, the tubes are swollen and inflamed. Movement of the cervix stretches the tubes and other tissue in patients with salpingitis or an infection in the tubes. In patients with appendicitis, this maneuver is seldom very painful. I asked the students, "What nerves are being stimulated by stretching the tubes?"

"The lumbosacral plexus," someone said.

"Does everyone agree? Okay. Now, the young woman in our case not only had severe pain and tenderness in both lower quadrants, she also had pain and tenderness in the right upper quadrant. And once she was placed in stirrups in preparation for her pelvic exam, she began to complain of pain in her right shoulder."

A student held up his hand. "Our case study text doesn't mention anything about pain in the shoulder," he said.

"I know it doesn't. I added the shoulder pain to make it more complicated. I want to see if you remember what you learned from your study of the thorax – the chest. But, tell me, how does the infection and pus get from the uterus into the abdominal – Peritoneal – cavity?"

Before he could respond, another student answered. "It travels through the tubes into the lower part of the abdominal cavity."

"Okay. Can you show me the point where the tubes end?"

"Do you mean the fimbriated end of the tube?"

"Yes. It looks like a wilted flower. There! You've got it," I said. "Now this infection irritates the lining of the abdominal cavity. What do you call the lining? Anybody?"

"Peritoneum," they all answered.

"And an infection of the peritoneum is called what?"

"Peritonitis," most replied.

"Okay. Let me remind you that this patient is tender in both lower quadrants. So where is the pus located?"

"In both lower quadrants," they answered in unison.

"Correct!" I continued. "She is also tender in the right upper quadrant. So where else is the pus?"

"The right upper quadrant," they all replied, smiling.

"You've got the picture. Okay!" I selected a young man who seemed reluctant to participate. "How does the pus get from the lower quadrant to the right upper quadrant?"

"It travels up the right colic gutter," he answered, moving his finger along the path.

"That's good. You know, you students are really smart. Now, when the pus gets to the right upper quadrant, it is located under the liver. What's that area called?"

"The hepatorenal pouch of Morrison," they sang out.

"Yeah, that's a mouthful, isn't it? But it's hard to forget. So, let's move on. The patient is lying flat on her back and her legs are up in the stirrups in preparation for the pelvic exam. She's complaining about pain in her right shoulder. Can anybody tell me what has happened?"

Nobody could, so I stood there shaking my head. "Oh, don't tell me you've all forgotten what you learned when we studied the chest. So let's review the anatomy of the phrenic nerve. Where does it come from?"

"From the neck," someone ventured.

"It does. And what does it do?"

"It moves the diaphragm during breathing."

"Does everyone agree with that?" I asked the group and they all nodded yes.

"Well, at least you remembered that much. I was going to throw cold water on anyone who didn't. Now the phrenic nerve also carries sensory pain fibers from several areas. What might they be?"

"The pleura," a student answered in a small voice.

"But what part of the pleura?"

"The pleura on top of the diaphragm." The student's voice was a little stronger now.

"What else?"

"The pleura lining the mediastinum."

"And what else?

"The covering of the heart – the pericardium."

"Brava! And that may be why some people with a heart attack get pain in the neck and shoulders. What else?" When no one knew the answer, I asked, "What is the nerve supply to the peritoneum on the under surface of the diaphragm?" After a long pause, one student asked if it could it be the phrenic nerve.

"You better believe it," I told him, "and when we study the head and neck you'll learn again that the phrenic nerve comes from the same spinal level as the nerves that carry sensation from the neck and shoulder. You see, our brain is unable to interpret the signal accurately. So an irritation of the heart, the pleura or the diaphragm is often interpreted as pain originating in the shoulder and neck. That's called 'referred pain.' We often call referred pain the soul of medicine – that's S-O-U-L soul. Now back to my question. What's happening to cause this patient to feel pain in her right shoulder?"

All the hands went up. "The pus is irritating the under surface of the diaphragm!"

"Great," I said. "Now you've all got it. So, listen up! I don't give a damn if you don't remember trivia like the nerve supply to the subclavius muscle. But, for the rest of your lives, remember this: any patient with an infection in the abdomen or pelvis who is also complaining of pain in the shoulder is a very sick patient! The patient probably has perforation of the bowel or the appendix and usually needs surgery urgently!"

I gave them a moment to let that sink in. "The only exception to that," I said, "is a case like the one we're discussing right now.

"This young woman showed up in the ER with pelvic inflammatory disease. It turned out that she was sexually active and had an IUD in place – an intrauterine device to protect her against unwanted pregnancy. Unfortunately, it didn't protect her from a sexually transmitted disease. Her male partner had gonorrheal uretheritis, commonly referred to as 'the clap.' He transmitted the infection to her. It began as an infection in her cervix and her cervical canal and it produced a yellow vaginal discharge. That kind of PID – pelvic inflammatory disease from gonorrhea – can generally be treated successfully with antibiotics alone."

One of the brightest students asked, "Wouldn't you also have a vaginal discharge in a patient whose appendix had ruptured?"

"That's a very good question. The answer is yes. But the pus would be a muddy color with a foul fecal smell due to multiple bacteria. The pus from gonorrhea is yellow and has a characteristic odor that is not offensive. Of course, the pus from a ruptured appendix or a perforated bowel can travel down the fallopian tubes and through the uterus causing a vaginal discharge. But a simple smear can identify the single bacterium – a single germ – in gonorrhea and the multiple bacteria in appendicitis. You'll learn a lot more about bacteria next year and then the clinical features of illness in your third year. But, right now, here's something to remember:

"If a vaginal discharge has a foul fecal smell to it, it can only come from a perforated bowel or appendix– or, more infrequently, a contaminated obstetrical procedure – a dirty abortion. You're all too young to remember what it was like 50 years ago when abortions were illegal. A lot of poor, desperate women died because of dirty coat hangers and knitting needles used on them by some quack or some lady down the street.

"Come to think of it," I said, "most of the people who want to ban all abortions today aren't old enough to remember those days, either. But, at any rate, the laws may change again and when you're doctors you may find yourself dealing with foul-smelling vaginal discharges caused by illegal abortionists, not perforated bowels. So be careful and don't jump to conclusions."

I had one last question for them about the woman with the IUD problem we had been discussing. "She recovered and left the hospital okay, but do you think she could have been spared a lot of trouble if her partner had used a condom? That's something you can talk about while you're eating your lunch."

I had my lunch in the faculty dining room, quite content to let the students argue among themselves without me. Americans seem to have made up their minds about the use of condoms for birth control or disease prevention and I doubt that any of those minds are about to be changed by anything that conflicts with their opinions or beliefs. All I can add to any discussion is my own experience over years, going back to my Army days at the military base in Rochefort, France.

SEVERAL MONTHS AFTER WE had cleaned up the red-light district in the town, the colonel commanding our post called an unscheduled conference of all unit commanders, including the chaplain and me.

"Gentlemen," Colonel Dann said, "we have a serious fucking problem on our hands – and I mean that literally!"

The other officers turned to look at me. I immediately thought that something must have gone terribly wrong at one of the Rochefort brothels – or maybe at all of them. But I was wrong.

The American Army had a central high school on our military base. It was a boarding school. The children of soldiers stationed in various posts throughout our region of France were bussed to our high school every Monday. During the week, the teenagers were with us. On Fridays, they were bussed home to be with their families for the weekend. The school's dormitory south wall faced the Charente River. And that's where the problem was discovered.

Maintenance crews had responded to complaints of sewage backing up into the first-floor lavatories. When they checked the main sewage pipe that carried waste to the river, they found it completely clogged. "Have you seen that pipe?" growled the colonel. "That damn pipe is big enough for a man to bend over and walk right through it! Can you imagine what plugged it up?"

He glared about the room at us. "*Rubbers*, Gentlemen! And I don't mean the kind you put on your feet! Hundreds of them! Maybe thousands! Completely clogging the sewer! Those horny little bastards must have been screwing their brains out for *years!*"

The chaplain looked stricken. The captains and lieutenants struggled to suppress any sign of amusement. The one major in the room, a by-the-book guy who wasn't the brightest spark on the post, volunteered that there would be dire consequences if this situation became public – or if the parents got wind of it. As usual, he had immediately grasped the obvious.

"So what are we going to do, Gentleman?" said the colonel. "We've got to keep a lid on this unless we want to be flooded with reporters and congressmen – not to mention the brass from Headquarters in Orleans. We're not their favorite people as it is."

The lieutenant who was the post public information officer spoke up. He had once worked for a newspaper in civilian life. "I can tell you from my own experience," he said, "that the press will go crazy over this story, if it gets out. As they say: it's got everything – from their point of view, of course, Sir. Do the kids know yet what we found in the sewer pipe?"

"No, they don't," said the captain in charge of maintenance. "We've kept everyone away from the work site. The only one we've told about what we found is the CO. So I have a suggestion. We'll have to close the dormitory anyway, until we dig up that sewer pipe and clean it out. So why not put the kids on busses and send them home to their folks. Tell 'em it's nothing more than something that happens to sewer pipes from time to time, but that it'll take us a while to fix it."

"But what do we tell the students when they come back?" said the colonel.

"We must separate the boys from the girls," said the dim-bulb major.

"They're already separated," snapped the colonel. "The boys live on the second floor; the girls live on the first floor. There are adult chaperones on both floors. Always have been. You'd think somebody would have noticed that much screwing going on for Lord-only-knows how many years. Anybody have any idea on how these kids are getting together?"

"I didn't think much of it at the time," said the Provost, "but a few months ago one of my MPs told me he'd caught a boy shimmying down a rope on the backside of the dormitory, the side by the river. The kid said he was just trying to sneak out of the dorm without being noticed. The MP gave him a warning and sent him back to his room. It never occurred to the MP – or me, either – that the kid might have been trying to reach some girl's window on the first floor."

"Well, I'll be damned! That's exactly how they do it! Shimmying down to the girls' rooms, having sex, flushing the used condoms down the toilets and then shimmying back upstairs. Okay, we send the kids home, and we search the dorm. I bet we find more than one length of rope hidden on the second floor. We'll make those ropes disappear."

"But, Colonel, if the boys can't find their ropes, won't they know that we know what they been doing?"

"Sure they will. So what? Maybe it'll throw the fear of God into them. Make 'em think twice before screwing around again. Any other ideas?"

There was no shortage of suggestions: from increasing the number of chaperones to making the isolated south side of the school dorm a regular nighttime MP patrol. The chaplain thought some lectures on abstinence might be helpful. Everyone seemed to agree that if we could put a stop to the sexual shenanigans, there'd be no need to make anything public about what had been going on.

"What about you, Doc?" said the colonel. "You haven't said a word about any of this."

"Getting rid of the ropes is a good idea," I said. "A kid could fall and break his neck, Sir."

The laughter Colonel Dann's officers had been suppressing erupted. When it subsided, I got serious. "I know teenagers, Colonel. They'll out-smart us sooner or later and start filling up another drainpipe. But I think we should thank our lucky stars that they've been smart enough to use condoms. Speaking as a doctor, I find that clogged sewer pipe sort of reassuring. I'm not aware that any female student has become pregnant here. And, as far as I can tell, no student – male or female – has contracted a venereal disease."

"Well, then," said the colonel. "Let's keep it that way."

I HAVE NO DATA to support any conclusions that might be drawn from the Rochefort school dormitory sewer-pipe-clogging affair. I'm not a moral theologian and I have no quarrel with abstinence. But, despite increased chaperones and military police patrols, I assume that the students found new ways to engage in sexual activity. They always do.

"Let your conscience be your guide," is a good admonition. But so is "Do no harm." Condoms do decrease the chances of a girl's getting pregnant, thus making it easier for her to say "Yes" rather than "No!" But unprotected sex greatly increases the risk for contracting a venereal disease. Condoms, some people argue, don't offer 100% protection and, therefore, shouldn't be used at all. But condoms do reduce risk significantly and are vastly better than nothing at all.

As a doctor, I was pleased with the way Colonel Dann handled the situation. He made it more difficult for the teenagers to get together to have sex, but he did nothing to cut off their supply of condoms. The Army, he often explained, wasn't in the business of encouraging or condoning immorality, but that didn't mean that the Army should facilitate stupidity.

7

HOW I LEARNED ABOUT WOMEN

SEVERAL TIMES A MONTH, I would receive phone calls from attorneys seeking advice about potential malpractice cases. I estimate that I got about 2,000 calls over 35 years. The merits of most of the cases (or the lack thereof) could be determined within a few minutes. The vast majority could be dismissed over the phone as lacking merit. For some, I would request the medical records for review. For a few of them, I would refer the lawyer to an appropriate specialist. But after one call, I invited the lawyer to come to my office to discuss a case in detail. It was a case in which a woman had lost a kidney following a hysterectomy. That was something I happened to know something about – thanks to another lucky break.

After two years in the Army, I returned to the United States to begin a residency in General Surgery at the Washington Hospital Center in the District of Columbia. Now most general surgeons, including those of my generation, have limited experience in gynecology. During their residency training, they spend a few months working with gynecologists. During that time, the general surgical resident may be allowed to do a few D & Cs for abnormal bleeding and remove one or two ovaries – and not much more beyond that. But on the first day of my rotation, the chief resident sat me down for an interview and, after she determined that I was someone she could trust, she told me her story.

The chief resident was married to a radiologist. She and her husband had been trying to have children without success for almost 20 years. When her periods stopped, she assumed that it was the beginning of menopause. She went on vacation with her husband to visit her family in Germany. While she was there, her old family physician examined her and gave her some startling news. She was not beginning menopause. After years of disappointment, she was going to have a baby.

"And here I am," she said. "I am in my forties and five months pregnant, as you can see. My husband and I are happy, of course, but I am finding that at my age I fatigue very easily. I desperately need my sleep at night. So, Dick, I have a proposition for you. If you will take for me all the emergency night calls in the ER and on the wards, I will let you do *all* the major cases."

"Wow!" I said. "Have you got a deal!"

I will be forever grateful to that woman who spent so much time training and teaching me. During those four months under her supervision, I seldom had an uninterrupted night's sleep; but I performed about 30 hysterectomies plus a dozen A&P repairs of fallen bladders and umpteen D&Cs. I handled two ectopic pregnancies, one tuboplasty and the removal of several ovarian cysts. I also acquired considerable experience in treating acute and chronic pelvic inflammatory disease due primarily to gonorrhea.

When I came to the Manhattan VA Hospital in 1964, I found that there were no gynecologists on the staff. So, for the next three years, all female surgical patients were placed on my ward so that I was able to teach general surgical residents how to perform D&Cs and hysterectomies. My ego got a real lift when an OR nurse who needed a hysterectomy asked me to do it.

DURING MY GYNECOLOGY TRAINING in Washington, I had been taught to make sure to protect a woman's ureter during surgery. The ureters are tubes connecting the kidneys to the bladder. They allow urine to flow to the bladder where it's stored until the woman urinates. Now, when I teach anatomy to first year students, I demonstrate on the cadaver how the ureter is in harm's way during removal of the uterus. "If you ever cut a ureter," I tell them, "you'll have to talk to your lawyer."

I've reviewed four malpractice cases where the ureters were accidentally cut or ligated. One occurred during a Caesarian section, one during a vaginal hysterectomy, one during an abdominal hysterectomy and one during resection of large bowel. One patient lost the function of a kidney. The other three recovered kidney function once the injured ureter was repaired. The ureter was never identified during any of these procedures although the surgeon who performed the colon resection had dictated in his operation report that the left ureter had been "identified and protected." Subsequent surgery revealed the distal end of the left ureter was missing. What the surgeon had "identified" was, in all probability, ovarian vessels.

FOR DOCTORS, SERIOUS CONSEQUENCES result from not knowing one's anatomy. Consider the median nerve injury during a surgeon's resection of a "synovial cyst" (ganglion) from the wrist. The patient was a middle-aged, right-handed woman who was referred to the general surgeon because of a tender lump on the front of the right wrist. The lump had been present for many years. As a child, she had sustained a small laceration in that area. The surgeon diagnosed "ganglion" or "synovial cyst" and opted to remove it in his office under local anesthesia.

After making a skin incision, he found a one-centimeter lump attached to what he thought was the Palmaris Longus tendon. He removed the lump along with a short segment of the "tendon." Then he repaired the "tendon" with a figure-eight wire suture – the Paul Bunnell stitch. The patient recalled that during the operation, her thumb and fingers had twitched violently on several occasions.

Following surgery, the patient had marked limitation in the movement of the thumb and numbness in the thumb, index, middle and half of the ring finger. It was obvious that she had median nerve palsy. The pathology report showed that the lump was a neuroma attached to a major peripheral nerve.

The Paul Bunnell wire suture technique is fine for a tendon repair, but it's a disaster for a nerve repair which requires very fine suturing technique on the surface of a nerve. A wire suture going in and out of the nerve in several places will destroy a long segment of a nerve. A subsequent attempt by a plastic hand surgeon to repair the damaged median nerve was unsuccessful because about two inches of the nerve had been destroyed by the wire suture used in the "tendon repair". Important parts of four fingers of the patient's right hand remained numb – the parts that we use for tactile dexterity. That rendered the woman's dominant hand almost useless.

Her case was settled without going to trial. Like most anatomical blunders, this one could have been avoided if the general surgeon had taken the time to look at an anatomy atlas before performing the operation.

SOMETHING ELSE I'VE NOTICED over the years is that some doctors have the problem of inordinate modesty or squeamishness when it comes to examining women. That, too, can have dire consequences.

In the autumn of 1963, just a few months after completing my four-year surgical residency, I entered the doctors' locker room at Tompkins County Hospital in Ithaca, NY, where I was starting my private practice. It was about 11 o'clock in the morning and I had just completed a radical abdominal perineal resection for a large cancer of the rectum. The patient was a middle-aged woman, a registered nurse.

As I was getting out of my scrubs and changing into my street clothes, another doctor walked into the locker room. I had met him before and liked him. He was highly regarded and an extremely capable internist and he wanted to ask me about the patient on whom I had just operated.

"How did it go, Dick?"

"Pretty easy and it went fast. It's always easier with a woman. They have a much larger pelvis to work in, as you know."

"Right," he said. "Was her liver clean?"

"As far as I could tell, it was. I couldn't see or feel any evidence of metastasis."

"Thank God for that," he said. "How about her lymph nodes?"

He wasn't just making small talk, I realized. The doctor was seriously concerned about this patient and I hated to give him the answer.

"I'm sorry, Fred. I suspect they'll be positive. I could feel several hard lumps in the mesentery."

"That's terrible," he said, almost to himself. "That's just awful. That really reduces her chances of a cure."

Yeah, I thought, it sure does: from 80 percent down to 25 percent. But all I could say was, "Sit down on the bench, Fred."

The doctor sank down and leaned his back against the lockers. "The woman you operated on," he said without looking up. "She's been my office nurse for years. My God, I feel just dreadful. She's like family."

He was trying hard not to cry, but remorse and pain welled up in his eyes. This wonderful doctor was being crushed by an enormous load of sorrow. And I didn't know what to do for him. He was older than I was: maybe twice my age. I wanted to comfort him, but the best I could do was to sit down beside him and say, "I'm so sorry, Fred."

"Dammit, dammit, dammit!" He banged his fist on his knee. "She was complaining of blood in her stool for over 18 months! For 18 months! And I just kept prescribing suppositories! I never did a rectal exam! Can you believe that? No rectal exam! Just goddam suppositories! I just can't believe I let it go!"

"Every doctor makes mistakes, Fred. Even very good doctors like yourself."

"Yeah, I know. But I'm going to live with this mistake for the rest of my life."

I couldn't think of anything to do except sit with him quietly until he regained his composure. That took a while. Finally, he wiped his eyes and stood up, weary and defeated.

"Well, thanks for everything, Dick," he said. "Please take good care of her."

"I will, Fred. You can count on that." I watched him walk to the locker room door and stand with his hand on the knob. "I can only hope that someday she'll find it in her heart to forgive me." He opened the door and slowly walked away down the hallway.

Did his nurse ever forgive him? I have no idea. I do know that she had an uneventful recovery from her surgery. But I don't know if she had been cured by the radical operation I had performed. The following spring, I left my private practice in Ithaca to begin my academic career in Manhattan and I lost touch with both of them.

OVER THE YEARS, I learned that what happened to that nurse in Ithaca was by no means a unique event. I'm aware of at least a dozen cases of rectal cancer where a diagnosis was well within reach of an examining finger. But the doctors involved delayed doing rectal exams or proctoscopies for as long as six months to two years, even though their patients continued to report that they were passing blood or mucus from the rectum. Many of those cases were handled over the phone with prescriptions for suppositories. Most were never litigated, although most should have been.

Malignant tumors are the second leading cause of death in this country. Some cancers, such as cancer of the lung, pancreas, esophagus, stomach and ovary, fail to produce symptoms until late in their development. In those areas, the cure rate is low. But the earlier a malignancy is diagnosed and treated, regardless of the location, the better the survival rate. What I always tried to impress upon the medical students who rotated through my surgical practice is that once a patient seeks medical advice, complaining of a specific symptom that could be caused by cancer, the doctor must proceed to perform certain diagnostic tests without delay. This is not the time for procrastination.

When a patient has such things as a persistent cough or trouble swallowing or blood per rectum or a lump in the breast, delay becomes serious malpractice. It is negligence for a doctor to deprive a patient of a chance for a cure by failing to respond quickly and correctly to the patient's complaint. Treating a symptom without looking for the cause gets doctors into a lot of trouble. More importantly, it's the patient who suffers the consequences like that doctor's nurse in Ithaca, New York, back in 1963.

ONE AUGUST AFTERNOON, I had just finished telling the nurse's story to a new batch of third-year NYU medical students. They were beginning their 12-week surgical rotation and I didn't know them very well yet. But I could see that the nurse's case had captured their attention and, as far as I could tell, had got them thinking.

"Now let's talk about the dangers of treating a persistent anemia with iron and B-12 shots without looking for the cause. That also gets doctors and patients into a good deal of trouble. Here's a case in point."

I told the students about a family practitioner who found that one of his patients, a 49-year-old woman, was anemic. He treated her with iron and B-12 shots. About two years later, the woman was hospitalized because of a rapid pulse. The hospital found that she had an overactive thyroid gland. During her hospitalization, tests showed that she also had severe iron deficiency anemia with hemoglobin of 7.4 and hematocrit of 22.9 with normal B_{12} levels and folic acid levels. "So what do you think about that?" I asked.

A young man at the far end of the table spoke up. "It seems like she has been losing iron from blood loss. Was she still menstruating?"

"No, she was post-menopausal."

"What about ulcers with bleeding?"

"No."

"Any black stools?" another student asked.

"What would that imply?"

"Old blood coming from the intestines."

"That's good thinking. But, no, she didn't give a history of black stools, bloody stools or mucus in her stools." I looked around the table. "So what tests do you want to do?"

"Bone marrow biopsy?"

"That's a very good idea and, in fact, the test was done. It showed absent iron stores. What does that tell you?"

"She's got severe iron deficiency anemia," said a young woman.

"Correct. Do you know why?"

She didn't know, but another student had a hunch. "How about her diet?" he said. "What kind of food was she eating?"

"A regular diet. Nothing unusual or harmful. So what do you want to do with her?"

"Give her iron?"

It was time for me to put a little pressure on this new group of students. "She's been getting iron and B_{12} for two damn years!" That got them sitting straight up in their chairs. "Where do you think all the hemoglobin and iron is going? Does anybody know?" Nobody answered and that puzzled me. "Have any of you people rotated through internal medicine yet?" The students shook their heads.

"Okay, that tells me you've had only limited exposure to gastroenterology; so let me explain what we're dealing with here. A persistent iron deficiency anemia should have a thorough gastrointestinal work-up. How do we do that? We pass a scope down the patient's throat to look at the esophagus, the stomach and the duodenum. Then we pass a scope up from below to look at the rectum and the large bowel. Finally, a small bowel series with barium allows us to take some pictures and evaluate the small bowel. And what are we looking for? We're looking for a cancer that is bleeding so slowly that the patient's stools appear to be normal. Is that clear?"

"Yes," said one young woman. "Is that what this woman's doctor did?"

"I'm afraid not. Neither did the hospital. Her family physician continued to see her on a regular basis and he continued to give her intramuscular injections of iron and B_{12}. After almost five years of that treatment, the woman showed up at a hospital with abdominal cramps and a large bowel obstruction. It turned out that it was caused by a huge cancer in the upper part of her rectum. The obstruction was so severe that it blew out her cecum. That necessitated the removal of the right half of her colon. Three weeks later, the tumor was removed from the recto-sigmoid area. As you can imagine, she was one sick lady for several months."

The students sat silently shaking their heads.

"Hang on, there's more" I said. "About three years later, the woman had another abdominal operation to resect recurrent cancer in the pelvis. The prognosis isn't good. She's probably going to die from this malignancy because some jerk failed to properly endoscope a persistent case of anemia."

I could see that the students were upset by my presentation, so I decided to give them some relief. "Just remember this case when you become doctors," I said to them. "If I ever hear that any of you has made that kind of mistake, I'll be the first one to show up in court to testify for the patient who's suing you. I'll tell the jury that I taught you to handle the case differently."

That got some chuckles from the group, so I went on. "Another area where doctors can create a disaster for their patients is cancer of the lungs." I placed a series of chest X-rays on the viewing box and asked the students to take a good look at the picture on the left. "It shows a round, solitary 'coin' lesion in the right middle lobe. It's shaped like a coin and it measures 1.3 centimeters in diameter. What do you want to do with this patient?"

"Does he have any symptoms?" a student asked.

"No, this lesion showed up on his chest X-ray during a routine physical examination. The man had no cancer symptoms. So, what do you do?"

"Could you just watch the lesion for a few months?" another student asked. "And observe any change?"

"Yes, you could," I said. "It's small and it has a smooth periphery, which also suggests that it may be benign. You could repeat the

X-ray in three to six months and see if there's any change. That would be acceptable. But, unfortunately, the radiologist who made this film failed to identify the lesion."

I pointed to the next picture. "This X-ray was taken two years later and again it was read as normal. Note that the lesion has not increased in size. It's still 1.3 centimeters."

"I can't believe a radiologist missed that," a young woman said. "How old was the patient?"

"He was 34 years old. Do you think that matters?"

"Well," she said, "cancer of the lung is unusual in that age group isn't it?"

"Yes, it is. And he was a non-smoker. But does that rule out cancer?"

"I guess not," she said.

"Why do you say that?"

"If it did rule it out, Dr. Kessler, you wouldn't have asked me the question."

The rest of the students waited for my reaction. "I see you guys are beginning to figure me out. Let's see how you do with the patient." The students laughed and relaxed a little.

"Okay," I said. "Let's get serious. I can't emphasize this enough. Cancer of the lung can be round, it can occur in non-smokers and it can occur in this age group. It may not increase in size for two years or more. The best chance for a cure is to remove the cancer early. That gives you a 60-to-65 percent chance of a cure."

I pointed again to the second X-ray. "Here we have a solitary nodule in the peripheral lung field. Is it malignant or is it benign? What tests can be done to investigate the nature of this nodule?" There were several answers: "Bronchoscopy." "Bronchial washings." "Lung biopsy." All good suggestions, but I kept prodding them. "Anything else?"

"What about a skin test for tuberculosis?"

"Sure, this could be healed tuberculosis."

Two students spoke at once, asking what the doctor in the case actually did.

"Nothing," I said. "He did absolutely nothing. Why? Because he got that negative X-ray report from the radiologist, remember?"

"Oh, yeah," a student sighed.

"Okay, it's a year and a half later. Once again, our man is having a regular check-up and another routine chest X-ray. Take a look at this third picture. Can you all see it? It shows that the 1.3 lesion is now 1.5 centimeters in diameter. It's bigger. So what do you do now?"

"It's got to be biopsied or something," a young man said.

"You're right," I told him. "But the man's doctor opted to watch it and get another X-ray in six months."

"Did the man have any symptoms at this point?" someone asked.

"No, he didn't. And, if you look at the fourth X-ray, which was taken six months later, you can see that lesion is still 1.5 centimeters. Does that rule out cancer?"

"I guess not," one student said. The others nodded in agreement. "Right, it doesn't rule it out. And not just because I asked the question. Look at this next X-ray. It was taken nine months later. It shows that the lesion has increased in size from 1.5 centimeters to a full two centimeters. Now, what needs to be done? Anyone?"

"It's got to come out!" a student said. "At the very least, the man needs a biopsy!"

Another student asked, "Does the man have any symptoms yet?"

"No, there were no symptoms at this point," I said. "And no biopsy either. Once again, the man's doctor did nothing. Absolutely nothing! So what happened? Two years after this examination, the man saw a different doctor. He was complaining of chest pain and back pain and . . . ."

I couldn't finish the sentence. I was interrupted by a number of agitated young medical students. "My God!" said one. "You must be kidding! You can't let a case like this disappear for two years! Where the hell did this happen?"

"It happened in New Jersey and no, I'm not kidding. By the time the man saw the new doctor, he had swollen glands in the neck, a large mass in the hilar region of the lung and metastasis to the bones and liver. He was placed on chemotherapy. But he was dead in six months. End of story."

I switched off the viewing box. The students settled down. "Here's what to remember about that case," I told them. "When you're confronted with a solitary nodule in the lung, you must not procrastinate. You must find out what it is – even if you have to open up the patient's chest and remove it."

The students were writing in their notebooks and I waited for them to finish.

"The last area I want to discuss with you today involves a lump in the breast and what to do about it. What does a breast cancer feel like?"

"A hard, irregular non-tender mass," a student volunteered.

"Very good. That's the classic description. Now, the patient we'll be talking about was a 53-year-old woman who went to see her doctor because of a lump in her left breast. Her doctor examined her and found a two-centimeter lump in the upper outer quadrant of the breast. An irregular hard non-tender lump. What does that sound like to you?"

"Cancer," all of the students answered.

"Absolutely! The doctor also found that the skin over the tumor appeared to be retracted or dimpled over the lump. What does that sound like?"

"Cancer!"

"Correct. There was also a one-centimeter lump in the woman's left axilla – her armpit. Now what does that sound like to you?"

A student responded quickly. "The cancer has spread to a lymph node."

"Correct," I said. "So what would you do now?"

"Get a biopsy!"

"Right," I said. "I agree with you. And I gather that we all agree that there's nothing terribly complicated about this woman's case, right? Even so, her doctor decided to get a mammogram. It was interpreted as 'normal.' Now what could that mean?"

"Maybe it's not cancer?" a student replied.

"Well, it might not be cancer," I said. "But does a 'normal' mammogram report rule out cancer? Think about it."

I let them sit in silence for a while before I commented. "You still need a biopsy in a case like this where the physical exam is so very typical of cancer. Remember that, in at least five percent of cases, mammography may fail to show a cancer. That's called a false negative result. Personally, I wouldn't have wasted the time and money for a mammogram in this woman's case."

All the students wanted to know what happened to the woman. "The woman's doctor notified her that the mammography report was negative and he didn't see her again for eleven months. How does that sit with you?"

"That's terrible," said a young woman. "Did the lump get bigger?"

"Of course, it got bigger!"

The young woman's eyes widened. "I'm sorry I snapped at you," I said quickly. "I'm not angry with you. I'm angry about the doctor. You see, during that eleven months, the lump in the woman's breast more than doubled in size and many more lumps developed in her. She underwent a mastectomy and all of the 27 nodes in her axilla were involved with the tumor from her breast."

I collected my notes and my X-ray pictures and prepared to leave. "I'm really sorry about letting my anger show," I told the students. "But it's hard to review a case like this. The tragic fact is that this woman's chances for a cure were drastically reduced by her doctor's poor judgment. If you're a doctor and you find a breast lump that feels like a cancer, you had better be aggressive and get a biopsy. That's it for today. See you all next week."

I got out of the conference room in a hurry before any of my new students had a chance to delay my departure with a question. They seemed like a pretty good bunch and it probably would be a pleasure to work with them during the coming weeks, but I had more than enough of them for one day. I just wanted to get out of the damn conference room and out of the hospital. I needed to sit down by myself and sort things out. I went to my office, checked my appointment book and saw that there was nothing to keep me from leaving early in search of a little peace and quiet. There was a quiet bar a few blocks away where they knew me well enough to leave me alone, and that's where I went.

Why the hell was I so testy today? Why had I snapped at a perfectly nice young woman who had asked a perfectly good question? And why, after so many years, was I still upset about what happened to that nurse in Ithaca? And why had I cut short that afternoon's conference with the new students when there was more I could have told them? I sat alone at the end of the bar, fiddling with my drink and thinking about what I could have said and when I could have said it.

I COULD HAVE TOLD my medical students that it often made no difference if a doctor's tardy investigation turned up a cancer that had already spread to the liver, lungs or bones. If you discovered large tumors that had been present for years, your delay in making a diagnosis wouldn't alter the outcome. Just because you found out what was going on inside a patient didn't mean that you had the power to prevent the patient's certain death. Yeah, I could have told them, doctors aren't gods. They can't forestall the inevitable. That would have given them something really depressing to think about.

But they wouldn't have to worry too much about lawsuits. No good lawyer would be dumb enough to pursue a case against a doctor who couldn't perform a miracle. The doctor's defense lawyers would mount a stiff fight and most likely win. "Sure," they'd tell the jury, "the doctor was probably negligent for not doing a rectal exam for six months, but what the hell difference did that make? If he had done the exam several months earlier, the patient wouldn't have lived any longer."

No, that would really be a frivolous case! You see, when it comes to medical malpractice, lawyers for the plaintiff work on contingency. And no lawyer can make money pursuing hopeless cases. They don't make any money unless they win. And if they lose, they're out their pre-trial expenses. That's why they consult guys like me. We tell them if they've got a case they can win, or not. But some lawyers have trouble hearing the word "no."

I drifted back a few years and began rehashing a case that a couple of brash young lawyers had presented to me for review. It had to do with a rare chordoma tumor in a man's neck which was invading the man's spine and adjacent vascular structures. The man wanted to sue his doctor because the doctor had prescribed antibiotics for neck pain for three months before he got X-rays that showed what was really going on. The patient's lawyers kept telling me, "It's a terrible case of negligence by the doctor! Imagine! Treating neck pain with antibiotics for three whole months!"

I told them that it had been ignorant, uninformed and negligent for the doctor to wait three months before getting an X-ray. "But legally it doesn't matter," I told them. "This patient is going to die because this tumor is incurable." But the lawyers kept insisting: "Our client just might have been cured if he had been treated three months sooner! We really think we have a smoking gun here!"

"Look, guys," I finally said to them. "You're talking medical nonsense. The only procedure that would cure this tumor is amputation of the head. You'd have to cut it off just above the shoulders and that procedure isn't tolerated very well by human beings. It might work with earthworms, but not humans." I thought that was pretty good.

"WHAT DID THE LAWYERS DO?" asked the bartender.

Jeez! How long had I been talking to him? I must have been giving the bartender my lecture. Or "thinking out loud." That might be a better way to put it.

"Well," I said, while trying to figure out what had just happened, "I have no idea what they did with the case. The only reason I remember it so well is because they never paid my fee for the consultation. A couple of no-good shysters, that's what they were."

"Yeah, they were," said the bartender. "Care for another?"

"Maybe next time," I said. "I think maybe I've had enough."

8

HOW MY ATTITUDES
GOT ADJUSTED

▭

LOOKING BACK, I WOULD have to say that my negative feelings about malpractice litigation changed in the autumn of 1970. At the time, my professional medical career was moving steadily forward and a good deal of my comfortable day-to-day life was on automatic pilot, so to speak, even the daily task of getting to work.

I had learned how to beat the traffic on my commute to Manhattan from my home in Bergen County, New Jersey. If I could cross the George Washington Bridge by 6:30 in the morning, I had it made. Traffic was light and I could cruise down the East Side on the FDR Drive, take the 23rd Street exit, drive a couple of blocks and turn into my hospital's parking lot and into the empty space reserved for me as a general surgeon who had a full-time position as the Assistant Chief of Surgery at the Manhattan Veterans Administration Hospital, not to mention being a man who didn't have to worry about finding a free parking spot in New York City. Life was good.

Surgeons start their days early with seven o'clock rounds to see their patients before going to the operating room. The residents perform most of the operations with an attending surgeon supervising them. That was an important part of my job, training young doctors to become surgeons. Three years before, in 1967, our hospital had become affiliated with New York University, so some members of the VA's medical staff had faculty appointments at NYU.

I had an unusual dual appointment as Assistant Professor of Surgery and Cell Biology. So I not only taught surgery to the residents and medical students, but I also taught anatomy to the first year medical school class. And, just to keep myself busy, I was actively involved in research.

A great deal of valuable research takes place in VA Hospitals. I had a particular interest in diseases of the liver and portal hypertension which is high blood pressure in the veins of the abdomen. Alcoholics are prone to this complication once their drinking causes cirrhosis of the liver. My research was done in cooperation with the Department of Gastroenterology and our conclusions usually found their way into medical journals so I found myself publishing two or three research articles a year.

MY COMFORTABLE LIFE was thrown off-track one autumn morning in 1970 in the hospital parking lot. I was inserting my ID card into the slot of the machine that opens the parking lot gate when I caught a glimpse of something white floating down from the sky. A newspaper, maybe? The barrier went up. I drove through the gateway, turned to the left and looked around for the falling white object that had caught my eye.

When I saw what it was, I slammed on the brakes and jumped out of my car. Close to the building, just outside the ambulance door to the morgue, I saw a body lying twisted out of shape on the pavement. I ran to help. The young man's body was quivering, but I knew that involuntary motions occur before the brain finally stops delivering signals to the muscles. No, the young man was dead and there was nothing I could do to help him.

He was an orthopedic patient, I could tell. He was wearing VA hospital pajamas and he had full casts on both legs. The white plaster was what I had seen when he plummeted from the hospital. I looked up and decided he must have fallen – or jumped – from the eighth floor. That's where the orthopedic floor was located.

It was very early in the morning, but I could hear people talking inside the morgue. I banged on the door. An attendant swung it open. I saw that my friend Ben was inside performing an autopsy.

The three of us got the young man's body onto a gurney and rolled it into the morgue before cars began filling up the parking lot.

"Is he dead?" asked Ben. He was a brilliant neurologist and neuropathologist, but I could see he was rattled.

"The fall had to kill him," I said. "But we'd better make sure."

"You seem pretty calm about this, Dick," he said as we looked for signs of life,

"When I was in the Army I had to go to a French morgue to identify the body of a young soldier. I'd given him a discharge physical the day before. He passed with flying colors. He went out on the town to celebrate the end of his military career that night. He got drunk and tried to fly off the roof of a hotel. The fall killed him, just like this guy."

"What's going to happen now?" Ben said.

"There'll be a Board of Inquiry to determine exactly what happened to our friend here and if anyone here at the hospital screwed up."

During the investigation, the Board of Inquiry interviewed Ben and the morgue attendant and me, but everything we could tell them was after the fact. What the Board learned from other people at the hospital was that the day before his death, the young man had attempted suicide. He jumped out of a second floor window, but only succeeded in breaking both legs. His legs were set and put into casts from the feet to the hips. Then he was moved to the orthopedic ward to recover.

In hindsight, that was a mistake. He should have been locked up in the psychiatric ward. The orthopedic ward was on the eighth floor and it didn't have any protective bars on the windows. It never occurred to anyone that any patient – even a suicidal patient – would be able to get out of bed with both legs in long casts, hobble across the ward, open a window and jump. But that's exactly what the young veteran had managed to do.

As for the doctor who sent the young man to the orthopedic ward rather than the psych ward, the Board of Inquiry admonished him and let it go at that. I don't think the family of the young man ever sued the hospital. I suppose that, if they had, they would have won their case. But I never thought much about that at the time. The legalities were none of my business. I put that sort of speculation out of my mind until the day my neurologist friend asked me for a favor.

BEN TOLD ME THAT for the past several years he had been reviewing potential medical malpractice cases for law firms and he needed my help. An interesting case had been sent to him for review, but it was outside of his area of expertise. It was, he said, a legitimate case of severe negligence and the lawyers needed the expert opinion of a surgeon. He was hoping that I would take a look at the file.

"No thanks," I told him. "Testifying against other doctors turns me off and I'd rather not get involved."

"But this doctor is a complete disaster, Dick."

"Look, Ben, all doctors make mistakes. I've made them myself: technical errors in the OR that had to be fixed, mistakes in diagnoses, being late in recognizing post-operative complications. Any surgeon who says he hasn't made mistakes is either a liar or isn't doing much surgery."

"Yeah, Dick, but I'm sure you were always trying to do the right thing. This guy took out a man's gall bladder and then disappeared for about a week. Post-op complications developed and the patient died."

"You've got to be kidding. Seven days? What the hell was he doing all that time?"

"The old fart was off flying his airplane, playing with his race horses and banging his mistress."

"Where did this happen?"

"Upstate in the Catskills. The doctor owned the hospital. He was chief cook and bottle washer. He ran the whole thing. The lawyers would be very grateful if you'd just look through the records and tell them if they've got a case. They just need some guidance. You won't have to testify. How about it?"

"Well, OK," I said. "Any surgeon who doesn't see his patient for a whole week after an operation ought to be taken out and shot."

So I picked up the medical records and paged through them. The more I read, the angrier I got. Following the removal of his gall bladder, the patient developed a fever and was given Tylenol and an antibiotic. His abdomen became bloated and he began vomiting. He was given Compazine to relieve the nausea and vomiting. Besides the usual post-operative pain in the incision, he began to experience hiccoughs and pain in the right shoulder, an ominous symptom. The pain medication was increased. His pulse rate and temperature went up. His urine output was not being recorded. He was not being given IV fluids, but he was given clear liquids to drink.

An X-ray of the abdomen showed dilated bowel. That suggested an ileus – an intestinal paralysis secondary to infection. The patient began sweating profusely and became disoriented. By phone, the doctor ordered a cool sponge bath for the high fever. The abdomen became more distended and the pain spread to all areas of the abdomen.

Finally, after being called repeatedly for seven days, the surgeon showed up at his hospital and saw the patient for the first time since the removal of his gall bladder. By this time, the patient was in a state of septic shock – low blood pressure secondary to severe infection – and his family insisted that he be transferred to a better hospital. He was taken to Mt. Sinai in Manhattan where he was resuscitated vigorously with IV fluids, potent antibiotics and operated on again.

During surgery, doctors discovered that the tie on the cystic duct had come loose and resulting bile leakage had caused bile peritonitis. An abscess, which had formed under the liver and diaphragm, had ruptured into the large bowel. At this point, stool spread throughout the abdomen. There was no way Mt. Sinai could have saved him. Despite a colostomy, drainage of the infection and insertion of a tube in the bile duct, the patient succumbed to infection and died within a month.

I knew that a tie can come off a cystic duct after an operation. It happens. But I also knew that a reliable surgeon would recognize the need to re-explore the abdomen in the first two-to-three days after surgery. Within that time, the bile duct can be drained or re-sutured. In most cases, the patient will make a full recovery.

But during this critical time, this surgeon had managed the post-operative days with telephone orders rather than seeing the patient in person on daily rounds as is required. He had been busy with his numerous extracurricular activities. As a result, I could see, his patient had died.

The widow had sued the surgeon for negligence. According to her attorney's notes, she was not the first person to sue the doctor. He had been sued so many times that he could no longer obtain malpractice insurance. His latest blunder and the threat of yet another forced him to close up shop and retire to Florida.

By the time I finished reviewing the record of this doctor's egregious negligence I was not only eager to testify against him, I was also ready to take command of a firing squad that would deal with him once and for all. I called the widow's attorneys and made an appointment to give them my report. I was still angry when I arrived at their offices a few days later. They said they had something to tell me, but I ignored them and immediately launched into my report.

"This patient's heart may have stopped in Mt. Sinai," I said, "but he died several times before that. He died once when he was not re-explored for the bloating and pain in his shoulder. He died again when the pain in his belly spread to all areas of his abdomen and he was not re-explored. He died again because he was being managed by telephone orders for eight days. Basically, this patient was being cared for by remote control! And I'll be more than happy to testify for you against his doctor."

I sat down at the conference table. The attorneys looked at each other, obviously taken aback by my dramatic performance. There had been, they told me, some important new developments while I had been reviewing the case. For one thing, the patient's widow had remarried. For another, the surgeon they intended to sue had died in Florida (of natural causes, I was sorry to learn, not by firing squad). They were settling out of court with the surgeon's estate for a paltry $45,000. I must confess that I felt let down.

I had put some time and effort into the case and I had been itching for a fight, I guess. But, as my feelings of righteous anger dissipated, I realized my time hadn't been wasted. I had learned a lot. What shocked me most about the outrageous case was that the lawyers had found it so difficult to find a surgeon willing to review the medical records, let alone testify. They asked me if they could call upon my services again someday. And I found myself telling them that, yes, they could.

They did send me some other cases to review and even referred me to other law firms. And so my name began to be mentioned throughout the legal profession in the eastern half of the country. And, over the years, I evaluated hundreds of cases, roughly 80 percent for plaintiffs and 20 percent for defendants.

What I came to believe because of what I learned in the autumn of 1970 is simply this: if a patient has been harmed by negligence or serious deviations from standard medical practice, the patient most certainly deserves honest representation and fair compensation. But if the health care providers have done nothing wrong, they also need to be protected.

My responsibility, I discovered, was to be available to review potential malpractice cases and to call them as I saw them. I'm glad I accepted that challenge. It made me a better teacher and a better doctor.

9

THE DANGER OF KILLING PAIN

IN MOST CASES, THE DIAGNOSIS of a medical illness is routine. With a careful history and physical exam, the correct diagnosis can be made 80% of the time before any diagnostic tests are performed. But the diagnosis in the remaining 20% is more of a challenge. It may require numerous tests and consultations with colleagues. The worst thing a doctor can do is to administer drugs that suppress the patient's symptoms. That makes the diagnosis more difficult.

This is especially true when dealing with patients who have abdominal pain of unknown cause. The progression of abdominal pain and a change in its location are important clues. A change in the abdominal physical exam may support the progression of an infection and the need for urgent surgical intervention. An increase in the pulse rate, temperature and white blood count will inform the physician that an infection is getting worse and the patient needs a surgical consultation – now!

It is dangerous to relieve the pain with strong narcotics until a diagnosis has been established and a decision made on the best way to treat the problem – medically or surgically. It is more difficult for a surgeon to evaluate an acute abdominal pain if the referring physician has given the patient narcotics for pain and antibiotics for an elevated temperature. By the time the surgeon sees the patient, the physical exam of the abdomen may be benign and unrevealing, leading the consulting surgeon to conclude there is no evidence of appendicitis or diverticulitis, etc.

Masking the symptoms – or signs of a disease process – creates a false sense of security, a sense that all is well when the disease may be progressing and getting worse.

It must be extremely embarrassing for a primary care physician to have to call the surgeon back in one or two days because the patient is obviously very sick with a perforated bowel that's spewing intestinal contents throughout the abdominal cavity.

Surgeons who are called to evaluate an abdomen should also review the medical record to see what medications have been given as well as the intake and output of fluids, lab data, and vital sign records of blood pressure, pulse, respiration and temperature.

It's also informative to review the nurses' notes. Frequently, nurses record information regarding changes in pain, vomiting, and other problems of which the referring physician may not be aware. If the consulting surgeon discovers that the patient has received narcotics for pain within four hours, it behooves the doctor to stop all pain meds and to come back to reevaluate the abdomen when the patient is not sedated. Over the years, I have tried to impress upon my medical students that masking symptoms with medication before making a diagnosis can be a fatal mistake.

DURING MY OWN TRAINING, I learned that a medical student or a young doctor could learn as much from a bad doctor as from a good one. Novices tend to remember the instances of substandard methods that led to bad results and they promise themselves never to repeat those same mistakes in their own practice of medicine. Fortunately for my students, the work I have done reviewing medical cases for attorneys has given me a filing cabinet full of horrible examples. On any given week, when I wanted a case history for the conference with my third-year medical students, I had a good supply of reports to look through. And so, once again on this particular week, I started with the first manila folder on the top of the pile.

R.K. was a 38-year-old man who was hit by a car and sustained a serious head injury. X-rays revealed a fracture of the nose and possible fracture of the skull in the region of the right temple. He was very alert and the vital signs of pulse and blood pressure were normal. He was admitted to the hospital for observation because he had been "stunned." He was placed on a regular ward at 9 p.m. By 10 p.m., he was complaining of a headache. The attending doctor was called and ordered Tylenol with Codeine (but did not see the patient). By 10:20 p.m., he was lethargic and was moved at this time to a neurology ward for closer observation. By 10:45 p.m., he vomited. The doctor is called and he ordered Compazine to relieve the vomiting. At 11 p.m., a neurology doctor is called who cancels all medication orders but does not go and see the patient. However, he does order an intravenous line be inserted. At midnight, the attending doctor does see the patient and realizes a neurosurgeon may be needed. By 12:25 a.m., the right pupil is dilated and the eye is turned outward and the patient is unresponsive and shows labored breathing. The neurosurgeon arrives at 12:45 a.m., gives a drug to reduce brain swelling and puts a tube down the patient's windpipe to control his breathing with a respirator. He takes the patient to the X-ray department where an X-ray of the arteries in the patient's head reveals he is bleeding (epidural hemorrhage from middle meningeal artery). Surgery does not begin until 3:20 a.m. because this small hospital is unable to mobilize the OR any faster. The surgeon opened the skull, evacuated the blood and controlled the bleeding artery. Unfortunately, the expanding blood clot caused so much brain damage that the patient died 3 weeks later.

There were some important lessons to be learned from that case. If a head injury is going to cause a problem because of bleeding inside the skull, patients experience a headache, followed by vomiting and a change in the level of consciousness. They will become lethargic and eventually comatose. The administration of narcotics or sedating tranquilizers will cloud the issue because they may cause lethargy and make it more difficult to evaluate any change in a patient's mental status.

Further, the patient in this case was being managed by remote control between 9:00 p.m. and Midnight. There is a 50% mortality rate from epidural hematomas. However, when managed like this case, one could anticipate a mortality rate close to 100%. The R.K. case was interesting, but not what I was looking for. I set file aside for another day and picked up the next manila folder.

J.H., *a 60-year-old female, saw her family doctor with a one-day history of right-sided abdominal pain and nausea. There was slight tenderness in the right upper quadrant, no muscle guarding or rebound tenderness. The temperature was 98.6° and the white blood count was borderline at 10.5 with a left shift. The doctor's first impression was gall bladder disease. He prescribed Tigan suppositories for nausea and advised her to call back if she got worse. He should have reexamined her 4-6 hours later. She called the doctor back five days later and stated that she was still ill with cramps and diarrhea. He suspected it was a gall bladder infection, prescribed the antibiotic Ampicilin and advised her that he would hospitalize her in two or three days if she did not get better. He should have examined her then, repeated the blood tests and obtained a surgical consult for a patient with persistent undiagnosed abdominal pain. Her illness continued and, three days later, he admitted her to the hospital by phone without seeing his patient. He ordered Keflex (antibiotic), Bentyl (sedative anti-spasmodic), Demerol (narcotic), Seconal (barbiturate sleeping pill) and Tagamet to reduce acid in the stomach. The admitting note made by the house physician indicated the woman's pain was severe and localized to the right lower quadrant. The next day, the woman felt better because of all the narcotics, sedation and antibiotics. The abdominal pain, however, now involved all areas of the abdomen. There was diffuse tenderness, guarding and rebound all over the abdomen. There was a tender fullness palpated on the right side on rectal exam. The family doctor decides to call a gynecology consult. The GYN consult saw the patient and was able to palpate a 6 x 8 centimeter mass on the right side of the pelvis. However, there was only slight tenderness in this area because she had been given Demerol (75 mg) for pain one hour before the gynecologist examined her. He thus concluded that she had an ovarian cyst rather than an abscess. The next day, the progress note indicated that she was better except that there was pain in the right lower quadrant and that muscle guarding persisted. The temperature and pulse were not elevated. That was because she was getting an antibiotic that was suppressing the symptoms and clinical features of an abdominal infection which was actually getting worse. The next day a large mass could be palpated in the right lower quadrant and the patient developed diarrhea.*

Still, the temperature and pulse were normal and the white blood count was only slightly elevated. The following day she was finally taken to the OR for a planned total abdominal hysterectomy. As soon as the gynecologist opened the abdomen through a transverse incision, he found pus, lots of pus. Pus was everywhere originating from a ruptured appendiceal abscess. He drained the abscess and irrigated the abdomen. He left the wound open because of the degree of contamination. He was unable to find the appendix because of the severe infection throughout the area. She developed a huge ventral hernia in the incision, which was repaired 2 ½ years later. Her appendix was removed at that time.

My notes reminded me that a jury had found the family doctor negligent for managing the case by phone for several days and masking the symptoms with drugs before a diagnosis was made. If the woman had been diagnosed and operated on in a timely fashion, I had concluded, she most probably would not have had the severe wound infection that caused the hernia and the need for a repair. The damages were small and she was awarded $60,000. That case wasn't exactly what I wanted. So I kept searching.

***S.C.** was a 47-year-old female who sustained burns on her back, chest, face and neck. She had skin grafting at two and three weeks following admission to a major burn center. On the 35th hospital day, she began to experience nausea, vomiting and abdominal pain plus a loss of appetite. She was administered a potent narcotic (Levo-Dromoran) twice that day to relieve pain. The next day, the doctors on the burn team noted abdominal pain, tenderness and distension. The white blood count increased from 9.8 to 24.8 with a marked left shift. That night the pain became severe and she was given two more doses of the narcotic. There was tenderness and muscle guarding in all four quadrants of the abdomen. She had been managed for three days by the burn team before an attending surgeon saw her. He quickly recognized the need for urgent exploratory surgery. A ruptured appendix was found with pus circulating throughout the abdomen. Despite being re-operated on twice during the next 3 weeks to drain pus, she died of infection.*

I thought about that case for a while. It certainly reinforced my belief that the medical profession had become so specialized that physicians in one specialty tended to forget the basic principles that apply to other specialties or other sub-specialties.

The physician members of this patient's burn team were all general surgeons or at least had some training in general surgery, yet they forgot two basic rules. First, abdominal pains that persist for more than six hours are usually of surgical import. Second, you do not mask the symptoms of an undiagnosed illness with excessive medication.

My notation added: "The attending surgeon should have been called two days earlier." That case settled for an undisclosed amount. I kept looking through files.

D.P. was a 44-year-old female who went to the E.R. because of abdominal pain of one day's duration. Her temperature was 99. She walked in a bent over position because of the pain. The abdomen was distended and there was diffuse tenderness but no rebound tenderness. Despite an elevated white blood count (14.0) with a marked increase in the neutrophils (left shift), a doctor diagnosed a probable viral syndrome and sent her home with a prescription for Erythromycin and Flagyl (both antibiotics) and Dolobid (an anti-inflammatory agent). All three of these drugs can mask or minimize the symptoms of an infection and should not be given to a patient with undiagnosed abdominal pain and are of no value to patients with a viral illness. D.P. returned to the E.R. the next day – the third day of abdominal pain. She was vomiting and sweating and unable to get comfortable on the stretcher. Her temperature was now normal (because of the antibiotics and anti-inflammatory drugs). Despite diffuse abdominal tenderness, another doctor diagnosed gastroenteritis and sent her home with a narcotic (Tylenol #3) to be added to her other medications. The next day, she saw her family physician who recognized an "acute abdomen" and the need for hospitalization. He requested a surgical consult who noted that she had diffuse abdominal tenderness, muscle guarding and very marked rebound tenderness. The patient was afraid to cough because it caused excruciating abdominal pain. Her walking in a bent over position, her rebound tenderness and her pain on coughing were all manifestations of spreading peritonitis. The temperature and pulse were elevated. The white blood count was up to 17.2. The surgical consult diagnosed diverticulitis (unusual in a 44-year-old woman) because tenderness was maximized in the lower left quadrant. He opted to treat her medically for the next eight days.

I leaned back in my chair. In retrospect, it would be easy to label the ER doctor and surgical consult as blithering idiots. (If people are truly stupid, they can't get into medical school, let alone graduate.) But these doctors were being misled by drugs that prevented them from fully appreciating the seriousness of her disease. Even the first E.R. doctor was misled because the patient had been taking penicillin for a week – for a common cold. Antibiotics have no place in the treatment of an uncomplicated cold in otherwise healthy patients. Nevertheless, the E.R. doctors could be faulted for ordering the masking drugs in the first place. And, after admission, the surgeon proceeded to drop the ball.

One day after D.P.'s admission, the abdominal X-rays showed an increasing amount of gas accumulating in paralyzed intestines. The next day, Saturday, she had pain in her left shoulder indicating that pus was irritating the under-surface of her diaphragm. The surgeon, who was now managing the case over the weekend by remote control, put in an order by phone for an ultrasound of the abdomen. The ultrasound, which was not done until Monday, showed a large abscess in the pelvis. Still, the surgeon did not operate for four more days.

I remembered that it was at this point in my case review that I concluded that the surgeon was grossly incompetent and needed to return to medical school for further training on the subject of peritonitis. The patient managed to survive her ruptured appendix despite her doctors. Her recovery took three months and required three major operations: to drain the intra-abdominal abscesses, to relieve intestinal obstruction and to repair her ventral hernia. With early surgery, it is most probable that these additional operations could have been avoided. The case settled.

THE NEXT FILE I LOOKED THROUGH contained the case of a 58-year-old female who went to the hospital with a flare-up of diverticulitis. This is an infection in the large intestine that begins in small pouches, called diverticulae, that develop in the wall of the bowel. The condition is sometimes referred to as "left-sided appendicitis." So long as the infection remains confined to the bowel, it can usually be treated with antibiotics. But if an abscess develops or perforation occurs, then surgery is ultimately mandatory. If an abscess forms, a mass can be felt or seen on a CT scan or an ultrasound. When free perforation occurs, the pain spreads from the lower left quadrant of the abdomen to other areas of the abdomen. Tenderness also involves more than just the left lower quadrant.

R.F. arrived at the hospital late at night, there was only tenderness to deep palpation in the left lower quadrant. She was given Demerol plus Vistaril for pain and started on an antibiotic. This was appropriate treatment for localized diverticulitis. By the next morning, the woman's abdomen had become distended, her temperature was 102, her pulse 128 and her white blood count had increased to 14.2 with a very marked left shift – an increase in the number of multinucleated white blood cells, indicative of infection. There was tenderness, guarding and rebound in both lower quadrants and her urine output was zero during the night. The patient had been vomiting since admission. The treating doctor felt she needed a surgical consult. (Most likely, the bowel had been perforated as a result of the spreading infection. That's the normal sequence of events.) The woman was given narcotics twice that day and the surgical consultation did not take place until the following day. By this time, the patient was weak; complaining of a lot more pain and no bowel sounds could be heard. There was now tenderness, guarding and rebound in both lower quadrants and the left upper quadrant. The spreading peritonitis was, in fact, advancing. But the surgeon was not impressed with the physical findings because the patient had received a dose of narcotics one hour before he saw her. The woman was given narcotics five times that day and the doctors opted to continue with non-operative treatment. That decision was made, in part, because the patient said she was feeling better. She got an even larger dose of narcotics four times that day. The next day (her fifth day in the hospital), the woman's pain had spread to include the right upper quadrant. Her urine output was zero again for one eight-hour shift. She was sweating and her respirations were 40 per minute (the normal rate is 15-20). An X-ray of the abdomen revealed a small bowel obstruction. The Bun was 60 and the creatinine was 4.7 indicating that her kidneys were failing.

My review notes said: "Patient is very dehydrated because she has been getting only about one half the amount of IV fluids that she needs." But the doctor's progress notes that day stated: "slow improvement." The nurses' notes were more revealing. They described the woman's zero urine output, her sweating and her rapid breathing plus the pain in the upper right quadrant. Their notes also mentioned that the woman's urine output did not increase after she had been given a diuretic to stimulate the kidneys. In addition to the nurses' notes, a lab report showed a very serious drop in the oxygen in the patient's blood (PO_2 53).

All of this information was reported to the doctors who, nevertheless, chose to treat the patient by remote control for about 10 hours. Seven out of seven sets of doctors' orders that night were made over the telephone. Finally, the woman was transferred to an ICU at 1:30 a.m. That's where she should have been from Day Two. On the afternoon of Day Six, the doctors finally operated on the patient. They found a perforation of a diverticulitis of the colon and stool all over the abdomen. The operative report describes "tremendous soilage," "tremendous inflammation" and "adhesions."

It was clear to me, when I first reviewed this woman's medical record, that the perforation and soilage had been present for several days. It most probably occurred on Day Two when the woman's pain, tenderness, guarding and rebound extended from the left side to involve the right lower quadrant.

The record showed that the diseased colon was removed and a colostomy created. The surgery was very difficult because of the extensive infection. Despite an intensive effort to treat this critically ill patient – including re-operation to drain an abscess in the abdomen – R.F. died one month later from multiple organ failure caused by severe sepsis.

The woman's doctors had been lulled into a false sense of security by narcotics and antibiotics that made her feel better sometimes. When the surgeon first saw the patient, he should have stopped the pain medication and re-examined the abdomen a few hours later. That simple act might have made it obvious that the resolution of the patient's problem lay in the OR.

The doctors were sued for the delay in performing surgery, masking of symptoms and gross mismanagement of intravenous fluid therapy. (During the first four days of hospitalization, the woman's urine output totaled a measly 1500, an amount equal to what should have been her daily output.) The doctors blamed the patient for the delay, stating that the woman initially had refused surgery. The family denied this and there were no notations in the record by any nurse or doctor to indicate the patient was refusing surgery. One of the defendants stated during his deposition that "she was too sick to be uncooperative."

The expert witness for the defense, a surgeon, stated under oath that there was no delay in surgery of a perforation of the bowel since it was his opinion that the bowel did not rupture until the night before the surgery. I felt that his statement was either a bold-faced lie or the opinion of an ill-informed idiot. Since I knew this witness personally as a nationally known authority on infections, I could not conclude that he was an idiot. At any rate, the case never reached trial because of some legal technicality. No one ever told me exactly what that might have been. All I was told was: "The doctors are off the hook."

Would the death of **R.F.** be a suitable case for the next conference with my third-year medical students? Her tragic story tempted me because it highlighted an important point. Doctors have been taught – and I always taught my residents and students – that a patient's refusal to follow orders or accept recommended treatment must be documented in the record at the time it occurs. Otherwise, no one will believe it when the incident is merely recalled at a later date. From a legal point of view, if it is not in the chart, it didn't happen. It's a simple matter of keeping one's own rear end fireproof. An interesting point, of course, but not one I wanted to make at the next conference.

I TOOK OFF MY GLASSES and rubbed my eyes. It was time to take a break and clear my mind. On my walk down the hall, I checked my mail box. Tucked in with the advertising brochures and inter-office memos was a letter from a law firm in Chicago informing me that a case I had helped them with had been settled amicably. They thanked me for my assistance and looked forward to working with me again in the near future. I would soon get a check for my services, I knew, but no personal satisfaction.

It had been one of those cases that really pissed me off. The doctors involved had treated an elderly lady very badly in several aspects of her care and it struck me that this particular case in Chicago had several good teaching points. So I went back to my office, pulled the chart and prepared a summary to present to my students the following day at our weekly conference. I decided to start with a short lecture.

10

TAKING A CASE TO CLASS

"THE USE OF NARCOTICS with abdominal pain has long been a controversial subject," I told the third-year medical students seated around the long table in front of me. Recent reports indicate that a small dose of narcotic does not interfere with the diagnostic process. This is probably true when done under the controlled circumstances seen in these studies where the ER physicians and consulting surgeons work as a team from the beginning.

"The patients in these studies were not managed by remote control nor were they sent home with an undiagnosed surgical abdomen or with a prescription for narcotics. Further, the diagnostic work-up was not clouded by adding other drugs like tranquilizers, barbiturates, sleeping pills or antibiotics to the regimen.

"There are still many physicians, including myself, who are skeptical of this risky display of compassion. I don't want you walking out of here today with the impression that pain relief is permissible before a diagnosis is made and that pain relief can be administered in all circumstances.

"Not true! There are good reasons for the old policy of withholding pain relief until a diagnosis is made. If it's going to be breached, the physicians in charge of the patient's care must exercise great caution and close supervision. That should be mandatory!

"Okay, this afternoon I'm going to give you a case to manage, step by step. As we go along, I want you to tell me what diagnostic possibilities you might consider, what diagnostic tests you would order and then give me your proposed treatment plan. We'll compare your theoretical case management with the management provided to a real patient by her actual treating physicians.

"As always, I want you to interrupt the presentation when you have a question, or need diagnostic information or feel her doctors were doing something wrong."

A brave student raised his hand. "Is this another one of your malpractice cases, Dr. Kessler?"

"Yes, it is," I responded. "Is that okay with you?"

"I remember the last one was really depressing."

"Yeah, it was. But that's the point of these exercises. I don't want you ever to forget what can happen if you mistreat a patient. So brace yourself. This is the case of a 62-year-old female who went to the E.R. at 12:30 a.m. with a 12-hour history of lower abdominal pain. Her pulse was 74 and her temperature and white blood count were only slightly elevated. She had been taking prednisone for phlebitis. What do you think so far?"

"Well, phlebitis is an inflammation of a vein and prednisone is a steroid," said the brave one. "Are steroids appropriate for phlebitis?"

"Not that I'm aware of," I said. "You'll find that steroids are used too often by the medical profession, despite the known side effects. Since you brought it up, what's a major problem that can result from prolonged use of steroids?"

"They can screw up the immune system," he replied. "That could make an infection more lethal and harder to diagnose."

"Correct! Patients on steroids may have a serious infection and yet the pulse, temperature and white blood count remain normal or only slightly elevated. As in the case at hand, for example. The ER doctor examined the patient and noted that there was tenderness and guarding in both lower quadrants. What do we mean by muscle guarding?"

"Rigidity of the muscles."

"That's correct. And what could possibly be causing the pain and tenderness in this patient?" I walked to the blackboard. "Let's make a list of our differential diagnoses."

"How about diverticulitis?" a young woman suggested.

"Okay, we'll make diverticulitis Number One. What is it?"

"An infection in the diverticulae of the large bowel," she said confidently.

"What are diverticulae?"

"Little sacs that project out through the wall of the bowel, usually the large bowel and they tend to develop in older people."

"Right on!" I said. "What else should we put on this list?"

"How about appendicitis?"

"Absolutely! But you don't have to be tentative. When we're making a list of possible causes of abdominal pain, appendicitis should probably never be lower than Number Two or Three." I looked down toward the far end of the table. "What else?"

"Gastroenteritis."

"Okay. Number Three is gastroenteritis." I wrote it on the board. "Do you think gastroenteritis would cause muscle guarding?"

"No, it wouldn't."

"That's right. That would be an unlikely possibility since there was no vomiting or diarrhea. The doctor who saw this patient considered two possibilities – Two and One on our list – appendicitis and diverticulitis. What should he have done then?"

"He should have done a rectal exam."

"Is that what you would have done?"

"You bet!"

"Why?"

"To see if there was any tenderness or mass on either side of the pelvis."

"Oh, boy, here we go again," sighed one of the male students. I ignored him.

"What else do you think we should do for this patient?"

"Admit her to the hospital?" said a young woman. "Start an IV and get a surgical consult?" said another.

"And would you kind-hearted ladies want to give the patient something to relieve her pain?"

"Well, just how bad is her pain?"

"Oh, not too bad, But it was bad enough to bring her to the hospital after midnight."

"Well," said the other young woman, "we've been taught that it's not a good idea to cloud the issue with narcotics. So I guess I wouldn't give her anything."

"She may have an infection," I said. "How about giving her some antibiotics?"

"Oh, no!" said the first young woman. "No antibiotics, for the same reason."

"Well, what do we all think about what actually happened? This patient was sent home with a prescription for narcotics and advised to return the following day for re-evaluation."

Ira the Mumbler shook his head. (There's always been a mumbler in every class I've taught.) "That's terrible!" he groaned. 'I'll bet this case gets really disgusting."

"Yeah," I said, "it gets worse."

"Who was this doctor anyway?"

"An intern just one month out of medical school."

"Well, even so, he should have known better," said the Mumbler. "I mean, we're just third-year students and we know better than to send a patient like that home. What happened to her?"

"She returned to the hospital the next day," I replied. "That was 48 hours after the onset of her abdominal pain, which was now worse. Her abdomen was distended, her temperature was 101 degrees and she had not been urinating. Can you account for the lack of urine?"

"She was dehydrated."

"Right on. Her white blood count was increasing. It was now 15.2 with a left shift. What do you think that meant?"

"She probably had an infection and the steroids she had been taking for phlebitis were not suppressing her body's reaction to the infection."

"You're right. The woman's abdomen was tender with guarding and rebound tenderness in both lower quadrants. Let me ask someone else." I pointed to one of the young women. "What does rebound tenderness mean?"

She didn't hesitate. "The pain is made worse when the doctor suddenly removes the examining hand from the abdomen."

"Yes, but what does that mean?" That stopped her and no one else around the table volunteered an answer.

"Okay," I said. "Here's something to remember. You're examining the patient's abdomen. You remove your examining hand – suddenly. That jars the patient's belly. If that jarring of the belly increases the patient's pain, that tells you that you may be dealing with peritonitis or an infection in the abdominal cavity.

"Let me give you another test. Ask the patient to cough. Rebound tenderness is demonstrated by an increase in abdominal pain when the patient coughs. Also, you can ask the patient to stand on tiptoes and then drop down hard on the heels. That may also increase the abdominal pain, another indication of rebound tenderness. So, if you do find rebound tenderness, what should you do?"

Several students chimed in: "Get a surgical consult!"

"Everyone agree?" I looked around the table. "Okay, it's unanimous. That's good. Unfortunately, that's not what happened in the case we're looking at.

"Remember: the woman had returned to the hospital the next day with more abdominal pain, her abdomen distended, and her temperature at 101 degrees. She had not been urinating and that told *us*, at least, that she was dehydrated. The family practitioner was called. He examined her and concluded that she might have appendicitis or diverticulitis. What was his plan for treatment? Admit her to the hospital, give her IV antibiotics and observe."

"Observe?" The Mumbler had stopped mumbling. In fact, his voice was now an octave higher than usual. "Observe for what?"

"Aha!" I said. "You're really concerned about this woman. What exactly are you concerned *about*?"

"She has an infection that is involving both lower quadrants, for crying out loud!"

"So what?" I asked him.

"Appendicitis begins in the right lower quadrant," he snapped back. "If her pain, tenderness and rebound have spread to include another area of the abdomen, it means her appendix has ruptured and needs to be removed immediately. Or as soon as possible, right?"

"That's correct. But let's suppose, on the other hand, that she has diverticulitis. How should *that* be managed?" I pointed at the young woman on the Mumbler's left.

"Well, diverticulitis can be treated with antibiotics," she told me.

"The patient's doctor gave her Kefzol. Is that okay?"

"It will help," she said, "but it won't cover all the bugs you expect to find with diverticulitis or appendicitis."

"What bacteria are you concerned about that might not be covered by Kefzol?"

"The anaerobic bacteria," she replied."

"What are anaerobic bacteria?" I ask.

"Bugs that thrive in the absence of oxygen."

"Such as?"

"Bacteroides."

"Right on! Is that a bad bug?"

Several of the students answered at once: "Yes!"

"How often do you find bacteroides in patients with appendicitis or diverticulitis?" I surveyed the table, but no answer was forthcoming. "Ninety-five percent of the time!" I said. "Let me ask you this. What causes the foul odor of the pus you find in cases of perforated appendicitis or diverticulitis?"

I waited. Again, there was no answer.

"Bacterioides!" I took off my glasses and rubbed my eyes. "What other bugs can be present in a case like this?"

"E. Coli!" the students answered in unison.

"And does E. Coli cause a bad odor?" The students all agreed that it did. "Wrong!" I said. "A pure culture of E. Coli is odorless.

Remember that. Now what would have been a better antibiotic to use for infections involving the bowels?"

"Carbenacillin."

"Why?"

"It covers just about everything."

"Correct." I looked at the Mumbler who was now completely involved. "What other regimen could be used?"

"I'd suggest triple coverage," said Ira, "with Ampicilin, Gentamycin and Clindamycin."

"That's right. But don't forget that you shouldn't use any antibiotics until you have a good idea of what you are dealing with. If it really was early diverticulitis in this case, antibiotics might have resolved her problem. Right?"

"Right," he replied, "but her pain was in both lower quadrants. So something was probably perforated."

"Correct," I said. "But here's what happened. The doctor continued to observe her for the next five days! During those five days, her pain got worse, the distension got worse, the tenderness got worse, the abdomen became hard and diarrhea developed. Why the diarrhea?" I looked around the table.

No one responded, so I answered my own question. "Pus in the belly." I wrote on the blackboard: *Pus in the belly can irritate the bowel and cause diarrhea.* I underlined the words, put down my chalk and asked if there were any more questions.

"About the doctor," one student finally said. "Did he think of getting an X-ray?"

"Not soon enough," I said. "On the fifth day after her admission, the patient got a Barium enema. The pictures failed to show diverticulitis, but they *did* demonstrate the presence of a mass pressing against the large bowel – the colon."

"So she must have had a ruptured appendix!"

"Most likely," I said. "So, at this point, what do you imagine the doctor wanted to do with his patient? How do you think he should have proceeded?"

I polled the students, one by one. "Operate." "Explore." "Open her up!" Those were the answers I got from third-year medical students. "It seems that we're in general agreement," I said. "So, let's see what the doctor did next."

I saw the Mumbler slump down in his chair. "You know what's coming next, don't you?" I said to him. "At this point in the case, the doctor left on his scheduled vacation." The students groaned. The Mumbler shook his head in disbelief.

"Not only that, he neglected to leave an order for a surgical consult. So, over the next several days, the woman's case was managed by the house staff. At one point, they changed the antibiotic to Claforan. Would that cover bacteroides?"

"No!" the students responded.

"The house staff also ordered an ultra sound. It revealed a large abscess in the lower abdomen. What would you do now?"

Most of the students raised their hands and I pointed to a young man at the far end of the table. "I'd operate," he said. "And I'd drain the abdomen and take out the appendix."

"Well, the house staff *did* request a surgical consult."

"Finally!" said one of the young women. "About time!"

"But they didn't tell the surgeon that it was urgent," I said. "And they didn't tell him that the woman's temperature was 103 degrees. So, not having been advised of any urgency, the surgeon didn't arrive to see the patient until the next day. He went to her ward, but she wasn't there. He was told that she'd been taken to the X-ray department."

"Did you say she was on a *ward?*" said a young man. "I hope you meant an ICU."

"No, she wasn't in the Intensive Care Unit. She had been managed on a regular ward ever since her admission to the hospital."

"That's terrible!"

"Well, it wasn't good, was it? But what would *you* have done if you were the surgeon and you'd just been told your patient had been taken to the X-ray department? Would you have gone there to see her?"

"Maybe not, if I had something else I had to attend to," he said. "But I certainly would have made arrangements to be notified the minute she got back to her bed so I could examine her."

I asked the students if they agreed and they all did.

"Well, the surgeon didn't do either of those things," I told them. "He just went home. He didn't see her until the next day."

The students just stared at me. The Mumbler turned to the young woman sitting next to him and said, "I told you it was going to get worse."

"And it did get worse, didn't it?" I said. "Those X-rays the surgeon didn't see before he went home revealed a lot of fluid in both lungs. Also, the woman's breathing rate was 40 per minute. What does that suggest to you?"

"Sounds like pulmonary edema," said a young woman. "She was experiencing heart failure on top of everything else. How much fluid was she getting?"

"Three to four quarts of IV fluids daily."

"But how much did she weigh?" she asked.

"She weighed 120 pounds. So how much would she need for her basic water requirement?"

"She'd need 1500 cc per day plus some extra for fever and vomiting."

"Yeah, that's right. Very good. About one and a half quarts a day." I turned to another student. "What's the best way to monitor the fluids in someone this critical?"

"Urine output and a Swan-ganz catheter."

"What's a Swan-ganz catheter?" I asked.

"It's a catheter placed in the pulmonary artery to measure pulmonary wedge pressures. Can I ask what the readings were in this patient?"

"The Swan-ganz catheter wasn't used."

"How about a central venous catheter?"

"Again, a CV catheter was not used."

"What were the blood gases?"

"PO2 was 51."

"Wow! She was in real trouble."

"So what did she need?" I asked the group.

"Oxygen," said one student.

"A diuretic to eliminate excessive fluid," said another.

"Digitalis to support the heart," said a third.

"All very good ideas," I told them. "And she received all that and got a little better. The following day the surgeon examined her and concluded she was too sick to operate on."

"Too sick? I can't believe he said that!" Even the most reticent students were expressing outrage. "She can't *survive* without an operation!"

"Later that day," I pressed on, "the woman's blood pressure and urine output began to fall and the pH in her blood was 7.19. What does this mean?"

"She's developed septic shock with metabolic acidosis."

"How do you want to treat the low pH?"

"Give her sodium bicarb and go to the OR."

"Not done," I told them. "That wasn't done."

"Then this lady didn't have a chance."

"Not one chance in Hell," I said. "She died half an hour later."

The room fell silent and several moments passed before anyone asked if an autopsy was done. "Oh, yeah," I said. "The autopsy revealed a perforated appendix with foul smelling pus in every crevice of the abdominal cavity and a huge abscess in her lower abdomen."

"How much did she weigh at autopsy?"

"140 pounds."

"So she gained 20 pounds in the hospital," a young man said. "Seems like she was overloaded."

"Probably," I said. "But it's hard to tell without proper monitoring."

"I hope her family sued," a young woman exclaimed, but then caught herself. "Sorry," she said. "I forgot you said that this was a malpractice case."

"Indeed it was," I said. "Another one of those 'frivolous lawsuits' the politicians are always yapping about. But we're not in law school now, are we? We're here to learn from other people's mistakes so we don't make them ourselves."

I tossed my stick of chalk to the Mumbler. "My friend, here," I told the class, "is now going up to the blackboard to help us list everything that you think was done wrong in this woman's case. I want you to tell me how, in your opinion, the doctors deviated from accepted medical standards. Just jot it down," I told the Mumbler. "Neatness doesn't count."

I stood aside and let the third-year medical students compile the list of mistakes they had observed. They worked loudly and quickly. As their list grew longer, it became obvious that I was not dealing with a bunch of English majors. There were astounding lapses in grammar, syntax and spelling, but I was pleased. Their patch-work indictment showed me that they'd learned a thing or two about the proper practice of medicine. Here's my edited version of what I was able to decipher when their list was finished:

1. *Not admitting her sooner.*
2. *Sent her home with narcotics before diagnosis was made.*
3. *Masked symptoms with narcotics and antibiotics.*
4. *No surgical consult on Day 1.*
5. *Used inappropriate antibiotics in case of peritonitis.*
6. *Didn't operate when presence of abscess obvious.*
7. *Mismanaged IV fluid therapy.*
8. *Didn't transfer her to ICU.*
9. *Didn't use CVP or Swan-ganz catheter.*

"THAT'S PRETTY GOOD WORK," I told the students. "But how about the doctor who left on vacation without calling another attending physician?"

The student at the blackboard, now fully recovered from his case of the mumbles, was fiddling with the stick of chalk. "I was going to make that Number Ten," he said, "but I couldn't figure out how to phrase it, exactly."

"Well, just put down something," I said. "Anything at all. Just so we'll all remember."

"Okay, Dr. Kessler, if you say so." Ira the Mumbler took his piece of chalk and wrote:

10. Schmuck!

11

IS THIS SURGERY NECESSARY?

O NE AUTUMN DAY IN 1992, while walking up First Avenue from the VA hospital to the NYU Medical School, I found myself wrestling with the details of a malpractice case I had been asked to review. The case involved a 79-year-old man who had poor circulation in his legs.

As I walked uptown past Bellevue Hospital, I saw one of my old surgical residents approaching from the opposite direction. He had become a vascular surgeon after completing his training in general surgery and he was just the kind of man I wanted to see. After we exchanged greetings and pleasantries, I asked him the question that had been bothering me.

"When did surgeons stop doing lumbar sympathectomies, Walter? I haven't done one myself in about 20 years."

"It's been at least 20 years," said Walter. "Back in the late 60's or early 70's, we realized that cutting the sympathetic nerves did nothing to improve the circulation in the deep tissues of the lower extremities. Why are you asking?"

"I've been reviewing the medical record of a 79-year-old man who underwent a lumbar sympathectomy for infected ulcers in the leg and foot in 1986."

"1986? That's ridiculous. The surgery was unnecessary and a complete waste of time. Is this one of your malpractice cases?"

"Yeah, I'm just about ready to write my report to the lawyers."

"But 1986 was six years ago. Doesn't the statute of limitation run out after two years or so?"

"It does," I said. "But, in this case, the statute didn't start to run until 1990. That's when they discovered that they'd left a surgical sponge in the patient which caused kidney damage."

"Oh, my God," he said. "A serious complication from an unnecessary operation. That's *really* disgusting. The bastards *should* be sued."

"Well, you're a vascular surgeon, Walter. Would you be interested in testifying in this case? It happened in North Carolina."

"No thanks," he replied without missing a beat. "I don't want to testify against other doctors. But I do have a question about the sponge count in your case. Did the record say it was correct?"

"Yes, absolutely. They counted the sponges before, during and after the operation. And all three times they said they accounted for all the sponges."

"Obviously someone couldn't count properly."

"That's right. And the hospital's already indicated that they're going to settle out of court. It's the surgeon who refuses to settle. He claims it's not his fault that the nurses gave him an erroneous sponge count."

"He's got a point there, I suppose," said Walter. "But, even so, a surgeon is supposed to inspect the operative area before closing the incision to make sure all the instruments and sponges have been removed from the patient."

"That's right."

"You know," Walter said, "it's really terrible when serious complications develop after an operation that was useless or not indicated. I hate to say it, but the only reason nowadays for doing a sympathectomy for impaired circulation of the deep tissues in a lower extremity is to collect a fee."

"I have another case in my file that's even worse than that one."

"The only thing worse would be that the patient died."

"That's exactly what happened. An elderly lady with infected bones in her feet due to poor circulation was scheduled for a lumbar sympathectomy. The surgeon operated without an assistant and without any blood prepared in advance for a transfusion if one became necessary."

"That's two mistakes right there," said Walter.

"But that's not all. The surgeon accidentally made a half-inch tear in the vena cava. I know that could happen to anybody working near a vein in the abdomen, even though it's a large vein. But this surgeon didn't know how to go about repairing it."

"He never heard about the little Dutch boy who stuck his finger in the dike and saved Holland?" said Walter. "First, you stick your finger in the vein to keep the blood from gushing out. Then you keep it there until a vascular surgeon arrives to help you."

"Not this guy. He tried to repair the hole in the vein himself and he panicked. Every time he exposed the tear to suture it, the patient lost huge quantities of blood. The woman never got a transfusion and she bled to death in the OR."

"That's terrible. She died from an unnecessary operation. When did this happen?"

"Back around 1980."

Walter checked his watch. "I've got to run, Dick. I've got to get to the OR to help with an aortic aneurysm. But I really hope you win your case."

I HADN'T REALLY THOUGHT I could enlist Walter as an expert witness, but it had been worth a try. Leaving a surgical sponge or instrument inside a patient is a serious error, but at least it's an understandable human error. Nobody does it on purpose. But performing an operation that's not indicated – or no longer considered to be beneficial – seemed to me to be a serious violation of the Hippocratic Oath.

Physicians who engaged in this sort of conduct, I told myself, should be stripped of their licenses to practice medicine or, at least, be seriously disciplined. Maybe drawn and quartered, I decided, just before I arrived at the medical school.

When I walked into the Anatomy lab, I saw that the students were beginning to dissect the necks of their cadavers. I went from table to table pointing out the spinal accessory nerve which, I reminded them, was very vulnerable to injury when a surgeon is removing a swollen gland or a lymph node from the side of the neck. Later, when they had finished their dissections, I gathered them together and emphasized the importance of protecting that nerve.

"I want to tell you about a young woman who went to see a surgeon because of a three-quarter-of-an-inch lump in the side of her neck. The surgeon wisely decided to wait and observe the lump before taking any action. One week later, the lump had shrunk to one-quarter-of-an-inch, which proved that it was the result of an infection and should be left alone. Nevertheless, two weeks later, the surgeon removed the node under local anesthesia.

"During that procedure, on at least two occasions, the young woman's left arm flew out of control. Following surgery, she developed a painful sagging shoulder, plus atrophy of the trapezius muscle on the side of her neck and a shoulder blade that stuck out of the back – a winged scapula. She was left with a cosmetic and functional defect that is permanent.

"The surgeon claimed that he removed the lump because it had become bigger. His claim was demolished by the pathology report, which showed that the lymph node he had removed was one-quarter inch in diameter. It had *not* enlarged.

"As far as I'm concerned," I told the students, "the surgeon's reasons for taking out the lump are irrelevant. Cutting the spinal accessory nerve by mistake was an unacceptable complication that careful dissection and a thorough knowledge of anatomy could have prevented. If one of you ever makes that mistake in the future, you'll have to talk to your lawyer."

There was some nervous laughter. There always is when I make that remark, but none when I point out to my students what I find most tragic about the young woman's case. "The tragedy," I tell them, "is that her operation wasn't necessary in the first place."

I LEFT THE ANATOMY LAB and found myself thinking about my old friend, the late Dr. David Faulkenstein. I suppose my memories were triggered by my failure to enlist my old student, the vascular surgeon, as an expert witness earlier that morning. In past years, whenever I needed the expertise of a gastroenterologist on a medical malpractice case, I frequently called upon Dave Faulkenstein and he was always willing to help.

He served as Chief of the GI Service at the Manhattan VA Hospital for several years before his untimely death from colon cancer. An outstanding clinician, teacher and researcher, he also reviewed medical records for law firms and we collaborated on a number of cases.

That afternoon I remembered, as if it were yesterday, going to his office to consult him about an esophageal motility problem in the presence of a stroke. I had been looking over a case of a 60-year-old woman who had her gallbladder removed because of the presence of gallstones. Two weeks later, she had a stroke. Her left side became partially paralyzed. The stroke also created an esophageal motility problem, making it difficult for her to swallow.

"That was dysphagia," said Dave. "Dysphagia is a common consequence of a stroke. It can be so severe that the patient may need to be fed through a tube. What else happened?"

"She continued to experience extreme difficulty in swallowing and that persisted off and on for the next two years. She was hospitalized for evaluation of the dysphagia and also the chest pains that had been occurring intermittently for many years. They looked down her esophagus with an endoscope and saw abnormal waves of muscle contractions in the esophagus and some reflux of stomach contents into the esophagus causing a mild irritation."

"Esophagitis," said Dave. "Reflux is a common condition in obese patients, especially if they smoke."

"Well, she was a smoker," I said. "She was five feet, six inches tall and she weighted 195 pounds."

"Okay. So how did they treat her?"

"They gave her a weight reduction diet and antacids."

"Any H-2 blockers such as Cimetidine?"

"No, but she got better without them."

"So, what's the problem, Dick?"

"Instead of continuing with medical treatment, which seemed to be working, she was operated on. She underwent a Nissen procedure to prevent reflux of stomach acids into the esophagus."

"A Nissen procedure? That's the worst goddam thing they could have done! You don't do that to a patient whose swallowing difficulty is tied to a stroke! Screwing around with her esophagus is going to make it worse! Where the hell did this happen?"

"Out in Chicago," I said. "And it *did* make her dysphagia worse. It also started a chain of events that literally put her through hell for the next four years."

"Are you going to tell me that she got the gas-bloat syndrome from the Nissen operation?"

"Yes, indeed," I said. "She couldn't belch or vomit and her abdomen became bloated and painful."

"What assholes!" Dave growled.

"Wait, there's more. When they did the Nissen operation, they inadvertently cut the two vagus nerves to the stomach so that its mobility was impaired. Now it took her stomach five hours to empty."

"Are you surgeons specifically trained to screw up your patients?"

"Look, Dave, it's a recognized complication, albeit an unacceptable one. A good surgeon will make sure that the vagus nerves are preserved."

"Yeah, yeah, yeah," said Dave. "So now the idiots had to enlarge the outlet to the stomach to improve gastric emptying, right?"

"You're right. They took her back to the OR and did a pyloroplasty."

"Did that help?"

"Her trouble swallowing continued and she developed a complication of the pyloroplasty."

"Don't tell me she got the Dumping Syndrome?"

"You got it right, Dave. After eating, she'd get abdominal cramps and diarrhea. swallowing was worse and she had gas, bloat and Dumping Syndrome. She was hospitalized six months later. The woman said then that she had been better off prior to surgery.

"There's a doctor's progress note that indicates that the Nissen procedure and pyloroplasty had been totally unsuccessful and that the motility problem in the esophagus was worse."

"Is that all?"

"Hell, no, it's just the beginning," I said, "She was taken back to the OR. The Nissen operation was undone and replaced with a Belsey procedure."

"Another operation to prevent reflux of stomach contents into the esophagus? Are you surgeons trained to believe that you're God and that you can fix every fucking problem with the scalpel? A Belsey operation is not going to help an esophageal motility problem. In fact, it may make it worse."

"Well, it didn't help," I said. "So six months later . . ."

"Oh, stop! Don't tell me those jokers did more surgery!"

"Yes, they did. And the more they operated, the worse it got. Six months later, they did a colon interposition utilizing a segment of large bowel and bringing it up into the chest between the stomach and upper end of the esophagus."

"Holy shit," said Dave. "That's terrible. And there's more, I guess."

"The hook-up between the colon and esophagus did not function well and acid refluxed from the stomach into the colon. Three months later, they performed an esophagectomy."

"They removed the woman's esophagus? That's outrageous lunacy!"

"And she didn't get better," I said. "Six months later, bile was refluxing into her stomach and colon. So they took her back to the OR where they removed the distal half of her stomach and created a Roux-y-gastro-jejunostomy."

"Disgusting," said Dave. "The only good thing about this case is that some surgical residents got exposed to a wide range of complicated surgical procedures."

"That's about right," I said. "It sure didn't help the woman's dysphagia. It persisted. Six months later, she was back in the OR for revision of the colon interposition with resection of part of her clavicle and her sternum. After the operation, she still had trouble swallowing. And she had a significant increase in her chest pain."

"No wonder, after they screwed around with her collar bone and her chest plate," said Dave. "I guess they were really proud of their great work."

"As a matter of fact," I said, "one of the surgeons went to a convention two weeks later and presented a paper on his experience with esophageal reflux. He included this woman's case in his presentation."

"Now, that's *chutzpah!*"

"Oh, yeah, and the surgeon went on to mention that one of his patients – actually the woman I've been telling you about – had developed severe post-operative dysphagia and had undergone a colon interposition and was currently doing well and was free of dysphagia."

"What a load of bullshit! Did the surgeon mention all the other syndromes and complicated operations that resulted from his surgical meddling?"

"No, he did not."

"I didn't think so. So what happened to the woman?"

"She continued to have severe trouble swallowing throughout the spring and summer and into the fall. That's when the surgeon's paper was published in a surgical journal. It still contained his gross misrepresentation of the facts of her case. So much for peer review."

"Did she get sent back to the OR again?"

"Yes, shortly after the surgeon returned from the meeting where he presented his paper. The woman's colon, which you remember was now in her chest, had kinked and needed to be revised. That was done and, one year later, they did a total gastrectomy to prevent reflux of bile into the stomach and colon."

"Good Lord, Dick! Here's a patient who's developed a serious motility problem in her esophagus after suffering a stroke. Instead of leaving her alone, as they should have, these doctors try to play God and make the patient worse. They complicate the problem with unnecessary surgery that contributes to years of misery. They shuttle her back and forth to the OR trying this, trying that, and achieving nothing but more misery for the poor woman. I truly hope this gets resolved before she dies."

"Well, that's the case her lawyers are going to argue," I said. "I'll let you know how it turns out."

"I can't get over that surgeon's paper," said Dave as he walked me to the door of his office. "I've known for years that a lot of crap gets published in American medical journals. But this takes the cake."

"Well," I said, "it's 'publish or perish,' as they say. That's how those of us in Academia climb the ladder. We all want to be promoted, don't we?"

"Aw, come on, Dick! We've published papers together and not one of ours was full of bull shit like that guy's paper!"

"I was being ironic, Dave. You know, when I was a resident, I had a mentor named Ted Winship. He'd been a prisoner of the Japanese during World War II and he hated the Japanese so much that he wouldn't let any of his residents refer to Hashimoto's Disease. 'It's chronic thyroiditis,' he'd say. 'Leave Hashimoto out of it!'

"Anyhow, when I met him, he was a well-published author on the pathology of the thyroid gland and he told me that up to 80 % of the papers in medical journals are nonsense."

"Oh, I agree," said Dave Faulkenstein. "And just think about how many tons of bull shit has been shoveled since you were a resident. Anyhow, be sure to let me know if that woman wins her case."

She did win, but it didn't help her much. Over the next two years, while her lawyers did their work, the woman developed severe malnutrition and bladder dysfunction. She suffered another stroke and could only be fed intravenously.

During his deposition, her surgeon claimed that he was not aware that the woman had suffered a stroke prior to her first operation. But, given the woman's medical history and her physical condition, he *should* have been aware. After all, when he first saw the 60-year-old, five-foot-six, 195-pound woman, she was partially paralyzed on one side.

The case was settled out of court a few months before the woman died. At the time of her death, she weighed less than 100 pounds.

THE UNNECESSARY SURGERY PROBLEM was never far from my mind when I was teaching. Whenever a new group of third-year medical students rotated through my surgical service at the VA hospital, I was required to give them a conference on the subject of hernias. I would always begin with a review of the anatomy of the inguinal region – the groin. I'd follow that with a discussion of the various surgical techniques used to repair a hernia and finish with a presentation of the complications observed in patients who have undergone hernia repair.

The repair of groin hernias is what doctors, if not their patients, regard as a "routine operation." Over the years, I've repaired, or helped young residents repair, two or three thousand inguinal hernias. That gives you an idea of how many groin hernias are repaired nationwide every year. For a general surgeon, they are "bread and butter." The operations pay the rent and they are relatively simple to perform. But they are not without risk.

That's a point I always tried to impress upon my students. One of the most disturbing complications to arise after groin surgery is the development of a neuroma on one of the nerves located in the operative field. A neuroma is a growth of nerve tissue that occurs on a nerve that has been bruised, stretched, cut or ligated with a suture. A surgeon is not culpable for the formation of a neuroma,

I told my students, unless it is due to inadvertent placement of a suture around a nerve.

A neuroma causes extreme pain in the groin. It is painful for the person to move. For some, even wearing clothes is painful. The pain can become so severe that the patient is labeled a "nut case" and referred to a psychiatrist.

Admittedly, chronic pain can make a person seem to be crazy. But the proper treatment is removal of the neuroma. I would end my groin hernia conferences by presenting a case of post-operative neuroma formation in a patient who underwent surgery that was unnecessary in the first place.

It's a case of a 28-year-old man who went to his doctor with a two-month history of pain in the left groin. The doctor examined the man and did not find a hernia in either groin. But, the doctor later stated, the man's external inguinal rings were enlarged on both sides.

Now enlarged external rings have not been considered clinically relevant since the 19th century, but this general-practice surgeon elected to operate based on an enlarged hole in the external oblique fascia.

The patient signed a consent form for a *left* inguinal hernia repair. The doctor operated on the *right* side. He explored the inguinal canal and found no hernia. He put in a few sutures to make the external ring smaller. After the surgery, he dictated his operative report describing what he found (nothing) and what he did (nothing).

When the patient woke up from the anesthesia, he asked the surgeon why the incision was on the right side. The surgeon, employing an excess of double-speak, told the patient that he decided to do the right side first since its ring was larger than the left side. He then re-dictated the operative report in an attempt to justify operating on the wrong side.

Two days later, this GP surgeon operated on the man's left side. He did not explore the inguinal canal but merely put in a few stitches to tighten the external ring. He billed the man for bilateral hernia repairs.

The man continued to have pain in his left groin. The pain was much worse and his groin was so tender that the doctor could not even examine him. So, five months later, the surgeon operated on the left groin again. This time he merely took out a few of the previous stitches making the external ring bigger. Again, he did not explore the inguinal canal.

The man still continued to have severe pain in his left groin. During the next two-and-a-half years, he went from doctor to doctor, from emergency room to emergency room, and from hospital to hospital because of the severe pain in his left groin and testicle. During this time, he was given narcotics for pain and underwent many diagnostic tests without success. He was even referred to a psychiatrist.

Eventually, he wound up in a university hospital where the doctors suspected that he had a neuroma – a lump of nerve tissue. They knew that there are two nerves that pass through the groin and exit through the external ring – the ileoinguinal and genitofemoral nerves. If one of these nerves becomes injured or sutured during an operation, a neuroma can develop and cause excruciating pain.

A university hospital surgeon explored the man's left inguinal canal and – sure enough – found a neuroma near the external ring. Four months later, the man developed the same problems in the right groin. During surgery, another neuroma was found and removed. Finally, this man was free of the terrible pain. The incompetent doctor who inflicted it on him settled out of court.

That case occurred almost 35 years ago, back in the days when some older doctors who had not had extensive surgical training were allowed to operate in small, non-teaching hospitals. Today, current hospital regulations prevent a poorly trained physician from setting foot in an OR. But, as I've always told my students, regulations are no defense against well-trained surgeons who have forgotten or ignored what they've been taught.

12

"CAN WE CHECK OUT THE OR?"

![decorative rule]

IT NEVER FAILS TO HAPPEN. Every school year, after the second or third week of classes, a few of the braver first-year medical students begin asking me if I could let them watch an operation at my hospital. Before long, almost all of their classmates get up the nerve to make the same request. It's been happening as long as I have been teaching anatomy. At first, I considered their requests to be premature; they were just starting their medical studies, after all. But, because they seemed serious and intensely curious, I said to myself: Why not? Inquisitive young minds need to be nurtured, not stifled, so after checking with the person in charge of the operating rooms, I began inviting them to come to the hospital, three at a time, to watch a surgical procedure from beginning to end.

NURSE VOLPE GREETED ME with a smile when I arrived at her office at 7:30 in the morning. Barbara Volpe was Supervisor of the Operating Room Suite at the Veterans Hospital in Manhattan and she ran the OR suite the way a good first sergeant in the U.S. Army runs an infantry company – firmly, fairly and efficiently. All of the VA surgeons knew that, without her commanding presence, we'd be lost. Barbara knew that we all knew who our Boss was really, but she was diplomatic enough never to rub it in. She was, as a matter of fact, the Authority I consulted on the possibility of student visits in the first place. Some Higher-Up signed the memo, but she was the one who gave the Okay.

"Your students are waiting for you in the locker room, Dr. Kessler," she told me. "They got here early, about half an hour ago, all bright-eyed and bushy-tailed. Two boys and a girl. They look real cute in their scrubs. I gave them the new ones."

"One side blue and the other side green?" I said. "The ones that make us look like clowns?"

"They're pretty popular," she said. "I'm having a hard time keeping them in stock."

"Well, I hear they make darn good pajamas, Barbara."

"So I gather. I've noticed that you've lifted a couple of pairs yourself, Doctor. Just don't wear them to the beach. People will stare. And please make sure your kids don't run off with my scrubs when they're finished today."

"Don't worry. I'll tell them."

I walked toward the locker room where my three students –Peggy, Howard and Tom – were trying to look calm, cool and collected. But they were obviously excited to be making their first visit to an operating room.

"I see Nurse Volpe has already outfitted you guys," I said. "Well, give me a minute to get into my scrubs and we'll go down the hall to OR Number Three. You'll be observing my residents doing a colon resection for cancer.

"And, by the way, Nurse Volpe wants me to remind you to return your scrubs to her when we're finished here. She's getting upset that they're disappearing so fast. I told her that medical students must be swiping them. So she's on the lookout for a fresh-faced scrubs thief."

"I hear she's pretty tough," said Howard.

"Oh, yeah," I said. "And she has a long memory. You don't want to get on her wrong side, that's for sure."

On the way to the OR, we stopped to watch my two surgical residents and a third-year medical student scrubbing their hands and arms. "They're prepping for surgery, I said. "It's a 10-to-15 minute procedure, removing as many bacteria as possible."

"Washing up takes a lot longer than it does in the movies," said Tom.

"So does everything," I said.

"Why do they need to do that when they're going to be wearing sterile gloves?"

"During surgery, rubber gloves frequently become torn or punctured. If you 'super clean' your hands – like they're doing now – you minimize the transfer of bacteria to the patient's surgical wound. So, everybody starts out as clean as can be, even the patient.

"A lot has already happened to our patient this morning, as you probably know, or may have experienced yourselves. An orderly washed the area of the patient's body that will be operated on. If necessary, the orderly shaved off any body hair in that area. He removed the patient's eyeglasses, dentures, wristwatch and jewelry – anything that could cause a problem during surgery.

"Then the patient was placed on a gurney and wheeled from his room to a waiting room adjacent to the OR. He probably got a mild sedative to alleviate any pre-op anxiety. When the OR was ready for the patient, his gurney was wheeled in and he was lifted onto the narrow operating table. If an electrical cautery was going to be used to control bleeding, a metal grounding plate would have been placed under him to prevent electrical burns."

We entered the OR and I told my students to stand close to the wall for a minute or two so that their eyes could get adjusted to the bright lights. Actually, I just wanted them to look around and soak up the atmosphere of the room. Also, I had some things to say that I didn't want the patient to hear – if he was still conscious. He was already on the table and the anesthesiologist was starting an IV in his arm.

"That's Dr. Z," I told my students. "She's a very skilled anesthesiologist, originally from Lithuania. I've worked with her at the head of the table hundreds of times and we've become pretty good friends. She'll answer any questions you may have. Not right now, but later, when she's not so busy. This is the way the OR is supposed to be at this point: a lot of hustle and bustle." The students watched as Dr. Z finished hooking up the IV.

"Right now," I said, "Dr. Z is the most important person in the room – besides the patient, of course. The IV she just started is a 'must' before a patient is put to sleep. It serves as the route by which she will administer the initial anesthetic agent that renders the patient unconscious. He's going to have general anesthesia, so she'll tape his eyes shut to prevent drying of the cornea. Now, during surgery, that IV line will serve as a route for administering IV solutions – or blood transfusions, if they should become necessary.

"See what she's doing now? She's using that sheet to secure the patient's arm and hand to his side. She's making sure that there won't be any pressure placed on his ulnar nerve. That's a nerve at the elbow, behind the funny bone. Also note how she's wrapping that sheet around his arm and tucking it under him. That's so his arm can't fall off the table. All that positioning is really important. Remind me to tell you more about it later."

Peggy, Howard and Tom watched Dr. Z applying electrocardiogram leads to the patient's chest. While she was doing that, the circulating nurse was putting pneumatic compression boots on the patient's legs.

"Those boots are very important," I said. "They've been a standard requirement since the late 1980s. They help prevent the formation of blood clots in the legs. Do you know about stasis?"

Tom answered promptly. "It's the slowing of the blood flow in the lower extremities. It may occur during periods of inactivity – like prolonged bed rest."

"That's right," I said. "And that can result in what we call 'deep vein thrombosis' – or DVT – which is clotting in the deep veins of the legs and thighs and even in the veins in the pelvis. If a clot breaks loose from those veins, it can travel to the heart and lungs. That causes a pulmonary embolism and the result can be a sudden fatality."

"Have you ever seen that happen?" Peggy asked.

"Oh, yes," I said, lowering my voice. "It's very frightening to watch someone die of a massive pulmonary embolism. They're okay one minute and the next minute they're anxious and short of breath. Then they start gasping for air and start turning blue. The veins in the neck stand out in bold relief. And, within minutes, they collapse and die."

"Just that suddenly? Without any warning? How can you expect a doctor to diagnose a problem when there aren't any symptoms?"

"You can't," I told her. "You just have to assume that a patient at risk for deep vein thrombosis may develop clots – like patients who are obese or have cancer, who are over 40 years old, patients who need pelvic or major orthopedic surgery, and any patient who's going to undergo surgery that will last longer than 30 minutes. And also, when you guys are operating yourselves, don't ever forget to use those boots on any patient who's been lying in bed for a long time."

"I didn't know that was such a serious problem in surgery," said Howard.

"Well, in surgical patients, the venous stasis and clot formation may begin on the operating table, once the patient is unconscious from the general anesthetic. And so you use prophylactic measures to reduce the incidence of pulmonary embolism.

"Also, I've seen studies that show that at least 30% of surgical patients develop deep vein thrombosis after an operation. DVT in the lower extremity may cause pain, tenderness and swelling of the extremity, especially calf tenderness. Most of these never cause a problem. But the studies suggest that over 50% of the surgical patients have no symptoms."

"How many people are we talking about, Dr. Kessler?"

"Approximately 150,000 people die each year of pulmonary embolism in the United States alone. That's in the general population. When it comes to surgical patients, you can greatly reduce the incidence of deep vein thrombosis and pulmonary embolism by applying those intermittent leg compression boots to prevent venous stasis. It's also helpful to give these patients low doses of the anti-clotting drug heparin. And these modalities, when needed, should be provided before, during and after surgery.

"Actually, it's now standard procedure to use these methods in patients who are at risk of developing DVT. So, failure to use the boots or the mini-heparin, or both, in high-risk patients can put the doctor in legal jeopardy if the patient dies of a pulmonary embolism."

"Wow," said Tom. "There's a lot to be careful about."

"Being careful is the name of the game," I said. "There's a lot that can go wrong in operating rooms, but most of it can be avoided. Take a look at what's happening now."

Two of the nurses were beginning their count of all the sponges, bandages and surgical instruments that had been brought into the OR. I moved my students closer to the operating area. I noticed that Tom's facemask had slid down exposing his nose and I reminded him to push it up so that his breath would be filtered through the gauze. Then I checked the man on the operating table. He was out cold.

"I want you to watch what Cynthia and Kathy are doing," I told my students. "It's extremely important. Those two nurses are counting everything on the tables that isn't nailed down. They count every item before the operation begins. They'll count them again halfway through the operation. They'll count them a third time after the surgery is completed. The numbers have to match each time."

"What if the numbers don't match?" asked Susan.

"It means that something's missing and they have to find it – whether it's a needle or an instrument or a gauze sponge. If it's on the floor or in the drapes covering the patient or in the trash bucket, it must be found and accounted for. If the incision has already been sutured and the object still hasn't been found, the abdomen must be X-rayed to make sure it isn't inside the patient. The patient must never leave the OR until the missing item is located."

"What if the nurses make a mistake in counting?" Howard asked.

"Then they have to own up to the mistake, right away," I said. "It's an extremely serious matter if the nurses state the sponge and instrument count is correct when, in fact, it is not. That's because missing objects inevitably surface weeks or months or years later inside patients. The missing object is discovered because it's caused a problem that no one had anticipated."

I saw that the nurses had finished their first count. "Cynthia," I asked, "when was the last time a sponge count was correct and the sponge was later found in a patient?"

"At this hospital, Dr. Kessler?" said the nurse. "It was about 20 years ago."

"What happened to the nurse involved?"

"She got fired. Barbara won't tolerate incorrect counts."

"You see, guys," I said to my students, "in the OR, you want to have nurses who are obsessive-compulsive about sponge and instrument counts. Sometimes they can drive a surgeon absolutely nuts. He's trying to complete an operation and they keep telling him that a sponge or hemostat is missing. Some surgeons are stubborn or arrogant enough to insist that the missing item can't be inside their patient.

"But I can't tell you how many times surgeons – and that includes me, myself – have been embarrassed when they finally explored their patient's abdomen and found the sponge or clamp or whatever it was the nurses said was missing. So, I say, God bless the top of the line OR nurses and their accurate sponge and instrument counts."

"So that really happens?" said Tom. "Stuff gets left inside the patient?"

"Much too often," I said. "And it's absolutely amazing how some objects found in the abdomen got there in the first place. I know of one hysterectomy case where a Balfour retractor was inadvertently left inside a woman."

"A Balfour Retractor?" said the Chief Surgical Resident from across the room. He was walking across the OR with his hands out in front of him, waiting for the scrub nurse to hand him a drying towel. "You've got to be kidding, Dr. Kessler! A Balfour is huge! Take a look," he said to my students. "We'll be using one in this operation. It's right over there."

The Balfour Retractor rested on the nurses' table, its folded stainless steel arms and blades reflecting the light from the powerful lamps shining down on the patient. Kathy, the nurse, held it up so that the students could get a good look.

"That's a really big instrument," said the Chief Surgical Resident. "It's got to be 10 by 5 by 4 inches when it's closed up like that. We use the Balfour to hold the bowels and the bladder away from the area where we're operating. And the retractor gets bigger when we open it up inside the patient. It gets to be about ten inches long and a foot wide! How the hell could anyone lose something like that?"

"Well," I said, "the patient was obese, well over 300 pounds. Somebody looked away for a minute, I guess, and the retractor just sank into the abdomen. Like it was sinking in quick sand, you might say. Then the layers of fat covered it up. The patient was obese, as I said, but that's a cop out. There's no excuse for losing a Balfour Retractor inside any patient."

"Amen to that," said the Chief Surgical Resident.

The Scrub Nurse, who handles all the sterile pads and instruments during the operation, slipped sterile surgical gloves onto the doctor's outstretched hands. The Circulating Nurse, who handles all the non-sterile materials and equipment in the OR, adjusted the doctor's surgical mask which now concealed his smile, but not the twinkle in his eyes.

"We're working with an audience today," he said to the nurses, "so I guess we'd better keep our eyes on the ball – and this Balfour Retractor."

I guided my students along the nurses' table and pointed out some of the smaller items that can sometimes go missing in the OR.

"Check out this little four-by-four-inch surgical sponge. It's used to blot up blood during a surgical procedure. Notice the blue thread that's woven into the fabric. The thread is radio opaque, meaning that it will show up on an X-ray. Sponges without that thread should never be used inside the abdomen or any other body cavity." I kept them moving along the table.

"Do you see that laparotomy pad over there? It's about the size of a dishtowel or a large washcloth? You'll see the assistant surgeon using one of those lap pads today to hold the bowels out of the way so that the surgeon-in-charge can see the organs he's working on.

"Notice that the lap pad has a long tail extending from one corner. The tail has a three-inch metal ring attached to it. You let the tail with the ring hang outside the incision. That's to remind the surgeon to remove the lap pad before closing up the patient. The ring must never be removed from the tail. Nor should the ring and tail be allowed to fall into the abdomen and disappear."

"How could anything that big just disappear into a belly?" asked Howard.

"Beats me," I said. "That Balfour Retractor did. And I know of several cases where a lap pad with a ring was left in the abdominal cavity. I know of some others where the lap pad didn't have a ring. I'll tell you about them later. Right now I want you to focus on the anesthesiologist. Is that Fentanyl you just gave him, Dr. Z?"

"Yes, it is," she answered.

"I remember getting Fentanyl just before my sinus operation," I said. "Let me tell you, it's the best damned euphoria you could ask for. Too bad it only lasted a few seconds before the lights went out." Everybody laughed except the unconscious patient.

"Okay," I said to my students, "Dr. Z has administered a muscle relaxant and now she's going to intubate the patient. Watch how carefully she inserts that tube. She's using a laryngoscope to look down the patient's throat. Once she sees the vocal cords, she'll pass the endotracheal tube between the cords into the trachea – the windpipe. I'm sure the students would appreciate seeing the vocal cords, Dr. Z, if that's possible?"

"Sure, this is an easy one," she said. Dr. Z leaned to one side so that each student could get a quick look. Then she passed the tube into the patient's trachea and began inflating his lungs with a mixture of air and extra oxygen. She used her stethoscope to listen to each side of the patient's chest.

"What she's doing now is extremely important. If the tube is in the right place, she'll be able to hear air going in and out of each lung. If she hears air going in and out of only the right lung – but not the left lung – the tube is in too far and has to be withdrawn until she can hear air going into both sides of the chest."

Dr. Z let one of the students listen with her stethoscope so that he could hear the air going into both lungs. Then she connected the endotracheal tube – the ET – to a respirator.

"What would it mean," Dr. Z asked the students, "if I failed to hear air going into either side of the chest? Well, it would mean that the tube is not in the trachea but has been passed down into the esophagus by mistake. I could confirm that by listening with a stethoscope applied to the upper abdomen. I would hear air gurgling in the stomach and that would tell me that the stomach would quickly become bloated. What would I have to do then?"

Dr. Z paused for dramatic effect and looked each student in the eye. "I would have to take the tube out immediately and repeat the process with the laryngoscope. And I would have to do it very quickly." Dr. Z turned back to her patient and I led the students away from the operating table so that I could talk to them without bothering her.

"Remember that I said the anesthesiologist is the most important member of the OR team at this point? When you come right down to it, it's almost impossible for a surgeon to kill a patient in the OR. The surgeon would have to commit some horrible screw-up or do something almost unheard of – like cutting a hole in something as important as the aorta or the heart. But an anesthesiologist or anesthetist, who doesn't do the job right, can kill a patient in a matter of minutes. Three minutes without oxygen will cause brain damage. Fifteen minutes without oxygen will stop the heart."

"Wow," said Tom. We turned our attention to the residents who were scrubbing the patient's abdomen with an antiseptic solution. I heard Tom whisper to Peggy, "What's an anesthetist?"

"That's a nurse trained in anesthesiology," she said. "An anesthesiologist is an MD."

"Oh, yeah," Tom said. "Thanks."

The OR nurses were draping the patient with sterile sheets. The operation was about to begin and it was time for me to leave the OR. "I'll see you later," I told my students. "Just stay here where you're not in anybody's way. Keep your eyes and ears open and do what the nurses tell you to do." Tom, Howard and Peggy nodded and looked back toward the operating table. Their eyes were fixed on the Chief Surgical Resident. "Okay, guys," I heard him say to the students as I walked to the OR door, "what you are going to be observing this morning is the removal of a cancerous sigmoid colon."

I SMILED TO MYSELF all the way to the OR office. The Chief Surgical Resident seemed confident about his ability to perform a successful operation and more than comfortable in his role as the star of this morning's show. My three young medical students were obviously thrilled to be in the presence of such an august being. He couldn't have asked for a better audience. There was enough paper work piled up on my desk to keep me busy until it was time to return to the OR.

I got there just as the Chief Resident was handing the circulating nurse the surgical specimen – two feet of the patient's large bowel. My three students were enthralled. I stood off to the side and watched them watching the surgical team sewing the two ends of bowel together. The operation was almost over and I was pleased to see that my students were switching their attention to the OR nurses who were finishing their third and final surgical-sponge-and-instrument count. One of the nurses reported that nothing was missing.

"Even the Balfour Retractor?" asked the Chief Resident.

"It's right here on the table," said Kathy.

"You're absolutely sure?"

"See for yourself, Doctor." Cynthia hoisted the bloodstained instrument off the table and held it up. "One Balfour Retractor, present and accounted for.

"Oh, thank God!" said the Chief Resident. "That's a relief! I guess we can close this guy up now."

He pointed to the third-year medical student who was playing a minor role in this operation. "Come over here, young man, and give us a hand. You're going to place some of these skin sutures for me." The Chief Surgical Resident had made the student's day. Mine, too.

I WAS RECALLING HOW I felt many years before when I was a medical student myself and was allowed to suture a laceration. And then I flashed forward to my days as an intern and a morning in 1956 at the Central Dispensary and Emergency Hospital in Washington, D.C.

That was the morning the Chief Surgical Resident handed me a scalpel and told me to make the first skin incision that would begin my first appendectomy. What a day that had been! The patient on the operating table before me was a 25-year-old physician from Argentina who was visiting relatives in Washington. He had come to our emergency room with a 24-hour history of pain in the right lower quadrant of his abdomen, a fever, an elevated white blood count and marked tenderness in the area of the appendix. Obviously appendicitis. Or so it seemed.

The Chief Surgical Resident who was supervising handed me a scalpel and said, "Go ahead, Dick." I took a deep breath and made my very first incision of a living human being – a classical McBurney incision in the right lower quadrant.

"Very good, Dick," the Chief Surgical Resident said to me. "I'll give you ten minutes to find the appendix. If you don't, I'll take over." I spent several minutes just trying to grasp the patient's slippery large bowel – the cecum. Finally I was able to push the cecum aside. There was the appendix, right where it was supposed to be – behind the cecum. But something was wrong!

"The appendix appears to be normal," I told the Chief Surgical Resident. "But take a look at that puddle of pus around the large bowel."

"Yeah, I see it, Dick. Looks like we have something more serious than appendicitis here. We're going to have to examine the small bowel."

"What are we looking for?

"Inflammation. Maybe he's got Crohn's disease – that's an inflammation of the small bowel – or maybe Meckel's Diverticulum."

We examined the small bowel carefully but found no abnormalities.

"So what do you think?"

"I have a hunch, Dick, but our incision's too small to let us examine his gall bladder and stomach. So we'll have to wait until we can. In the meantime, we'll send his appendix to Pathology and he'll have some diagnostic tests: an upper G.I. series – that sort of thing. Go ahead and take out his appendix and close him up. That's all we can do for him today."

"So it was a wrong diagnosis?"

"Yeah, I guess you could say that. But it got us this far. Now we know we have to keep looking beyond what his symptoms told us. That's something that happens: ten percent of the time in men and 20 percent of the time in women."

We got the Pathology report the next day. The appendix was indeed normal. The diagnostic test results revealed that the 25-year-old doctor had a lethal form of stomach cancer called *linitis plastica* or "leather-bottle" stomach – a type of malignancy rarely cured then or now. There was nothing that could be done for him and he went home to Argentina to die.

I LET GO OF MY REVERIE and focused on my students. The operation was over. The patient's wound had been sutured and the dressing applied. The Chief Surgical Resident was calling on Tom and Harold and Peggy to help lift the patient from the operating table to a bed.

"Be firm, but gentle," he was telling them. "He's not awake yet and he still has that endotracheal tube in place. Watch out for Dr. Z. Don't bump into her. She'll be supporting his head and neck while we move him."

"Yes, be careful," said the anesthesiologist. "And be careful while we're rolling his bed down the hall to the recovery room. I'll be breathing for him with this ambulatory bag attached to the endotracheal tube. His respiration must never be interrupted for more than a few seconds. So let's concentrate on what we're doing."

"Okay," said the Chief Surgical Resident. "Everybody ready? One, two, three, LIFT!"

Tom, Harold, Peggy and I followed the bed as the orderly rolled it slowly and carefully out of the OR and down the hospital corridor. Dr. Z walked by the side of the bed squeezing the ambulatory bag and making sure the patient was breathing properly. By the time our procession arrived at the recovery room, the patient was starting to open his eyes.

The orderly rolled the bed smoothly into its position against the recovery room wall. The patient coughed. Clearly, he didn't like the tube in this windpipe. Dr. Z removed it and the patient began breathing on his own. The recovery room nurse took over.

"I'm going to be monitoring the patient's pulse, blood pressure, urine output and respirations," the RR nurse told my students. "This little gadget that I'm attaching to the tip of our patient's index finger measures the oxygen saturation in his blood. It's called an oxymeter. When I first started here in the RR – and that was long before any of you were born – we had to estimate how much oxygen a patient was receiving. And we did that by observing the color of the patient's skin or fingernail beds. But nowadays this oxymeter can tell us if the patient isn't getting enough oxygen. We don't have to wait until a patient starts turning blue."

She patted the patient on his shoulder. "I'm just kidding, Charlie," she said. "You're coming along just fine." I knew Charlie. He'd fought in Korea and wasn't easily frightened. He smiled at the RR nurse and nodded. He was still pretty groggy, but he was coming around.

"Modern technology has certainly revolutionized our recovery rooms," I told the students, "but oxymeters and devices that measure blood gases can't replace the eyes and ears of the recovery room nurses. They have to stay alert."

"That's right," said the nurse. "Modern instruments can tell you a lot, but not everything. One thing we have to watch out for is hypoventilation. That's when the patient is breathing, but not deeply enough.

"Hypoventilation is one of the biggest dangers for a patient coming out of surgery and recovering from the effects of anesthetic drugs. If you don't quickly recognize the signs of hypoventilation, the patient will slowly become anoxic from insufficient oxygen. Also, the shallow respirations will fail to blow off carbon dioxide from the blood into the air. If you don't recognize hypoventilation and treat it immediately, it can lead to a cardiac arrest." She patted Charlie on the shoulder again. "But you're doing fine," she told him.

Howard wanted to know how a recovery room nurse would recognize hypoventilation.

"That's where experience makes a difference," she said. "You see that the patient is not wide awake. He's lethargic and his respirations are very shallow. He's unable to take a deep breath or follow commands. You know from experience that this is a dangerous situation that demands close observation and the measurement of blood gases. If you see that the patient is retaining CO_2, he needs to be re-intubated and put on a respirator for a while."

The nurse adjusted her patient's pillow. "But we're not talking about you, Charlie, are we? You're not having that problem. You're looking around the room and you're beginning to talk."

"Those kids," mumbled Charlie. "Who the hell are they?"

"They're first-year medical students. They're just starting their studies. Dr. Kessler wanted them to watch your operation."

Charlie stared at my three young students for a moment. "Well, how about that?" he said. "Did you kids learn anything?"

"Yes, sir," said Tom. "We learned a lot. And thank you very much."

"You're welcome," said Charlie. "Glad to help."

"Well, as you can see," Dr. Z said to my students, "our patient here did not have the problem we've been discussing. He's becoming more and more aware of his surroundings. He's not only talking, he's making perfect sense. The nurses will keep a close eye on him. But he's OK. No hypoventilation crisis for you to observe, thank goodness."

"Sorry about that," said Charlie. "I'll try to do better next time."

"See what I mean?" said Dr. Z. "Charlie's back to his old gruff self and I can go back to the OR. Why don't you take your students to lunch?"

"Good idea," I said. "Will you guys join me for lunch as my guests?"

"Of course they will," said Dr. Z. "Medical students never turn down a free meal. At least, none I've ever met. Neither do interns. I'll join you as soon as I can."

"Don't rush," I said. "We're going to stop by my office first and look at some X-ray pictures that show why sponge-and-instrument counts are so important."

13

LOST & FOUND
(INSIDE THE PATIENT)

▭

WALKING ALONG THE CORRIDOR to my office, I asked my students if they remembered the laparotomy pads I had shown them in the OR. "Yes," said Peggy. "They were about the size of big wash cloths."

"And they had metal rings in their tails," said Howard.

"Right," I said. "Well, I once reviewed the case of a 30-year-old female who had a Caesarean section. Five months later, she began experiencing nausea, vomiting, weight loss and abdominal pain. She was diagnosed and hospitalized for a bowel obstruction. Her X-rays revealed a foreign body in the right lower quadrant of her abdomen. It was a laparotomy pad, which had eroded into her small bowel.

"She had surgery, of course. The lap pad was removed and the hole in her bowel was sutured. But she developed a large incisional hernia which was repaired two years later using a mesh. The wound became infected and had to be debrided. But a chronic draining sinus with a foul odor persisted. I reviewed the OR records of her Caesarian section. They indicated to me that the nurses had probably not counted the sponges.

"Furthermore, sometime during the operation, the surgeon had removed the metal ring from the lap pad. That's something you should never do. The jury awarded the plaintiff $5,800,000."

"That's ridiculous!" said Howard. "Way too much!"

"I thought so," I said. "And the woman's attorney thought so, too. She said that it would probably be reduced to about $750,000, which is what they wanted in the first place. And it was. On appeal, the judgment was reduced by five million – down to $800,000.

That happens a lot. Outrageous jury awards usually get reduced on appeal."

Once the students were settled in my office, I put the film up on an X-ray view box and turned on the light. "What you're looking at is a post-operative X-ray of a 57-year-old woman who had a radical cystectomy. That's the removal of a urinary bladder because of cancer. At the same time, she had a hysterectomy and her surgeon created a new bladder from a segment of her bowel. Post-op, she developed gas pains, abdominal distention and abdominal tenderness. The X-rays I'm showing you were obtained nine days after her surgery. What do you see?"

"Well, I can see a tube going into the belly," Tom said, pointing at the X-ray.

"There's another tube here," said Howard.

"And another one here in the area of the kidney," said Peggy.

"You've got sharp eyes. Those tubes are in the ureters and they're draining into the new bladder."

"But, oh-oh!" said Peggy. "Look at that big ring there!"

"Bingo!" I said. "At least three doctors at the hospital looked at these pictures after the woman's surgery – the urologist who performed the operation, the general surgeon who participated and the radiologist. Would you believe that every one of them failed to spot this large ring? Or, if they did, they failed to identify it as a laparotomy pad marker. It was staring them right in the face as they reviewed the film and they failed to recognize it."

"You've got to be kidding!" said Howard. 'I can see the ring from where I'm standing way over here. And all three of us knew what it was right away."

"Yeah, it's pretty obvious," I said. "Well, the pad was eventually removed, but not before it created so much infection that the patient developed pulmonary embolisms that required a vena caval filter. It caused a breakdown of the hook-up between the ureters and the new bladder and that eventually necessitated a complete revision of the new bladder."

"What a mess," said Peggy. "And all because the OR nurses hadn't counted the lap pads correctly."

"And also because the urologist had made the mistake of allowing the ring attached to the lap pad to get into the woman's abdominal cavity during her initial surgery. As you've learned today, the ring is supposed to remain outside of the patient's body."

"There was a lawsuit?" asked Tom.

"Yes," I said, "but the case was settled during trial. That didn't help the patient much. She died of cancer two years later."

I put away the X-ray films and turned off the light in the viewing box. "Let's go to lunch," I said. The elevator took us down to the cafeteria on the second floor. We went through the serving line, made our selections and took our trays to a table in a far corner where we'd be able to talk undisturbed.

"Remember when we were back in the OR and I pointed out how carefully the patient's arm and hand were secured? So that there would be no pressure on his ulnar nerve?"

"Yes," said Howard. "You told us that the ulnar nerve was in the elbow behind the funny bone. But we haven't studied it in class yet."

"Then you don't know how many muscles in the hand the ulnar nerve controls. So I'll tell you. The answer is 14 muscles." I held up my right hand and flexed my fingers. "These little muscles are crucial for the dexterity that our fingers need to write or pick up objects. So we have to be careful not to injure the ulnar nerve in the OR. That can result in permanent ulnar nerve palsy. The hand becomes deformed into the shape of a claw and is partly numb – like this. As you can see, it's a very serious condition, especially in a dominant hand.

"I once reviewed a case of a 15-year-old boy who went to the hospital to have his tonsils and adenoids removed. He left with permanent ulnar nerve palsy to his right hand – his dominant hand. So remember, it's the responsibility of the OR nurse or the anesthesiologist to see to it that this type of injury can't occur.

"But when I reviewed the boy's OR record, I saw that his arms had been positioned at his sides. So how could he have sustained ulnar nerve palsy? His arm had either dropped off the side of the table or he had been positioned in such a way that his 'funny bone' was pressed against the table."

"Did anyone get sued for that?" asked Tom.

"You better believe it! That was what lawyers call a *res ipsa loquitor* case. That means that the case essentially speaks for itself."

Dr. Z sat down at our table. "I'm back," she said.

"And just in time. We're discussing how to avoid causing permanent ulnar nerve palsy in the OR."

"What about arm-boards?" asked Peggy. "We didn't see one, but couldn't they prevent that kind of injury?"

"Maybe, if they're used properly," I said. "If an arm is to be placed on an arm-board, the angle should not exceed 45 degrees. Consider this case. A middle-aged man enters the hospital for repair of a groin hernia and leaves with ulnar nerve palsy. Why? His arm had been placed on an arm-board at a right angle to the OR table – 90 degrees. That resulted in a stretch injury to the medial cord of the brachial plexus in the axilla."

I stuck out my left arm and pointed out the location of the injury. "Right here," I said, "in what you call the arm pit. In a few weeks, you'll be calling it the axilla."

"You'll be amazed at how your vocabularies will expand," said Dr. Z. "And you'll soon know all about medial cords and brachial plexi."

"But for now," I continued, "all you need to know is that the damage caused by this stretch injury was permanent. It involved most of the small muscles in the hand with a claw deformity. That case wound up in litigation and went to trial."

"I've seen many cases where the arm board was at 90 degrees and nothing happened to the hand," said Dr. Z.

"That's true," I said. "We get away with our mistakes most of the time. But when we don't, we have to talk to a lawyer."

"Point well taken," said Dr. Z. "Yes, it's better to do things correctly and not trust to luck that no harm will be done. But, speaking of lawsuits, have you ever seen a doctor sued because he or she failed to use pneumatic compression boots on a patient's legs?"

"Yes, indeed, several times. As a matter of fact, I just reviewed such a case. A 55-year-old man underwent an emergency colostomy because his colon was accidentally perforated by a colonoscope. Twelve days later, closure of the colostomy was performed. And one day after that, he died from a massive embolism that had originated from a thigh vein. He had not shown any symptoms or signs of a deep vein thrombosis. And neither pneumatic boots nor mini-heparin was used for either operation.

"The surgeons involved both testified that they liked to use the compression boots on all their cases. But they said that, on the days in question, the hospital did not have enough boots to go around for each operating room. This deflected some of the responsibility to the hospital and the hospital's insurance carrier."

"Did the doctors win?" asked Howard.

"Hell, no," I said. "The case settled halfway through trial. I know of another case of another middle-aged man who *did* show evidence of DVT before surgery – pain, swelling and tenderness in one leg. But his doctors ignored this. They operated on his colon without treating the DVT with heparin or inserting a filter into the inferior vena cava. The man died of a massive pulmonary embolism one day after colon surgery."

"There's absolutely no excuse for that," said Dr. Z. "It's not that difficult to do it right."

"Not difficult at all," I said. "We all saw how smoothly Charlie's operation went this morning. He was being managed properly with compression boots. And he'll be getting mini-heparin also."

"But can't heparin increase the risk of bleeding before and during surgery?" asked Peggy.

"That's an excellent question," I told her. "In general surgery, the risk is small and the advantages far outweigh the risk. However, heparin should never be used in eye surgery or neurosurgery where even the smallest amount of post-operative bleeding could be catastrophic.

"I know about a chief of surgery who testified under oath that he stopped using mini-heparin years ago because of post-operative bleeding. He also testified that if DVT was confined to the calf, he would just watch the patient. What a lot of nonsense! No wonder he'd been sued more than a dozen times."

When Dr. Z finished her lunch we got rid of our trays and returned to the table to continue our informal seminar.

"Having you three here today," I said, "and watching Dr. Z working with the patient, made me think about how many advances have been made in medicine since I was your age. When I was a student back in the 1950's, the field of anesthesia, for example, was still very primitive.

"The anesthesiologist checked the patient's pulse by feeling the temporal artery in front of the ear. Blood pressure was measured manually with a cuff on the arm. The heartbeat was monitored by a stethoscope taped to the front of the chest. And the anesthetic was administered by mask rather than through the endotracheal tube you saw Dr. Z inserting today. I remember administering open-drop ether onto a facemask. Of course, anybody who can remember that sort of thing is getting on in years. But, back in those days, one in 500 patients died on the OR table, primarily because of lousy anesthesia."

"He's right," said Dr. Z. "I remember those days. We did the best we could and hoped for the best."

"I know it's hard for you to imagine," I told the students, "but during an operation back then, the anesthesiologist was kept busy squeezing the bag that delivered oxygen and the anesthetic agent. The patient's pulse and blood pressure were recorded only occasionally – not constantly as they are today. Blood gas measurement devices and pulse oxymeters to measure oxygen saturation were not available in those days. But today you saw the pulse oxymeter on the patient's finger and the black boxes that recorded Charlie's heart rate and blood pressure automatically."

"Back then," said Dr. Z, "there was no way to know that your patient wasn't receiving enough oxygen until you saw the blood pressure and pulse numbers become abnormal. Or if you saw the patient turning blue. By which time, it was often too late."

"Sometimes," I said, "it would be the surgeon who first detected anoxia. He'd notice that the blood in the operative field had become very dark because of low oxygen. Worse yet, he'd become aware of the anoxia when he couldn't feel a pulse in the patient's aorta.

"The very first time I ever testified in court as an expert witness was in a case involving a 16-year-old female who had developed acute appendicitis. Before surgery, she was put to sleep with Pentothal. She was maintained on cyclopropane gas which was administered by mask—not an endotracheal tube. Twenty minutes into the appendectomy, the anesthesiologist announced that the girl had no pulse or blood pressure. The surgeon pulled back the drapes and saw that the patient's face was blue.

"All hell broke loose, as you can imagine. External cardiac massage, 100% oxygen, an injection of adrenalin into her heart. The girl was resuscitated and the surgeon was able to complete the operation. But the relatively short time that girl spent without adequate oxygen left her with severe and permanent brain damage. She was transferred to a nursing home where she spent the next 15 years of her life. The girl's mother visited her every day, but not once did her daughter ever recognize her."

"That's awful," said Dr. Z. "When did this happen?"

"In 1969," I replied.

"But endotracheal intubation was standard policy in 1969!"

"Not in that hospital. I was told that more than 200 appendectomies were performed there during 1969 and that endotracheal intubation had been used in only about 50 of those cases. The standard for that hospital was anesthesia administered by mask. The jury awarded the girl's family $2,000,000. That was reduced on appeal in 1974 to somewhere in the neighborhood of $800,000. Even so, that was a record for Chicago at the time."

"What's the risk in anesthesia today?" asked Tom.

"I think it is about one in 2,000. Isn't that about right, Dr. Z?"

"Maybe one in 1,500 to 2,000 cases," she answered. "Today, mask anesthesia is only used for brief operations that take no longer than five to ten minutes."

"But bad stuff still happens," I said. "I never thought I'd see another case like the Chicago girl's in 1969. But I was wrong. I reviewed a case that took place in 1989 – 20 years later!

"An elderly diabetic man was taken to an OR for amputation of a gangrenous toe and drainage of an infected foot. They put him to sleep with nitrous oxide and ethrane – by mask. When the drapes were removed after this 30-minute operation, the surgeon found that patient was blue and he had no pulse. A pulse oxymeter had been used. It was still on the man's finger. But it had malfunctioned. The old man was resuscitated, but he never regained consciousness. He died seven weeks later."

"Did you testify, Dr. Kessler?" asked Howard.

"No, I didn't. After I reviewed the case records, I advised the plaintiff's attorney that he would need an anesthesiologist to serve as the expert witness."

"Well," said Tom, "I understand about the risks of anesthesia by mask. But what about the risk when you're doing it right, with an endotracheal tube?"

"Good question," I said, "and more to the point about what you observed today during Charlie's operation. Let me tell you about another case. A 45-year-old man was taken to the OR to have incision and drainage of a Pilonidal abscess – that's an abscess on the butt. Doesn't sound like a complicated procedure, does it? But the nurse anesthetist did an endotracheal intubation and did not – I repeat – did not listen to the lungs after inserting the tube."

"Oh, my God!" said Dr. Z.

"The man's blood pressure and pulse were normal when the anesthesia was initiated. Twenty minutes later, he was turned over and the surgery on his buttocks began. Within ten minutes, the man's pulse was up to 120. Five minutes after that, his blood pressure was down to 92/50 and the surgeon noticed that the blood in the incision was very dark.

"Five minutes later, the patient was turned over. He was dead and could not be resuscitated. When the coroner did an autopsy, he concluded that death was due to natural causes."

"What crap!" Dr. Z, who rarely used profanity, leaned over to me and growled, "Did you see the autopsy report?"

"Yes, I did. The autopsy showed significant trauma in the right main-stem bronchus."

"There you go!" said Dr. Z. "The endotracheal tube had been inserted too far and had been passed into the right branch of the trachea so that only a portion of the right lung was being inflated. If the anesthetist had listened to the chest with a stethoscope when the tube was being inserted into the windpipe, she would have recognized the mistake and corrected it by drawing the tube up a few inches.

"You learned that this morning," Dr. Z said to the students. "You also learned that if the tube has been inserted into the esophagus by mistake, the patient's lungs will not be receiving any oxygen. That will kill the patient within 15-to-20 minutes if the problem isn't corrected. You're first-year medical students and already you know more than that coroner!"

"That's right," I said. "When we dissect a cadaver's neck in the anatomy lab, you'll see."

I got up from the table and went to the counter where they kept the silverware. I found two straws – one white and one with blue stripes. "Now we don't have to open anybody up," I said as I sat back down with the students.

"See this white straw? Let's say it's your trachea. Take a deep breath. Feel it? The air is going down your trachea or, in plain English, your windpipe. This straw with blue stripes is your esophagus. Swallow and see how it feels. The esophagus is the tube that the food goes down to your stomach and the trachea is the tube that air goes down to your lungs."

I put the two straws next to each other on the tabletop. "They're both inside your neck and they're pretty close together. And the vocal cords are in that area, too. You'll see just how close in the anatomy lab, but you get the idea, right?"

The students nodded and I went on. "I know of at least three cases where there was a cardiac arrest about 15 minutes after the start of anesthesia because the endotracheal tube was in the esophagus. That was gross malpractice. But not one of the cases was ever litigated. In fact, the families never even suspected that someone had mismanaged the anesthesia and caused the death of their loved ones."

"There's another major problem anesthesiologists are confronted with that you should know about," Dr. Z said to the students. "Remember when you looked through my laryngoscope and saw Charlie's vocal cords? Well, when it comes to the intubation of a patient who is obese with a short, fat neck, it's extremely difficult to extend the neck and lift up the larynx with the laryngoscope to view the vocal cords. Very often it's impossible to see the cords, so you have to pass the tube blindly through the nose into the trachea. Whenever we have a patient like that, we anticipate trouble. So we have two anesthesiologists on the case to help each other. If one can't pass the endotracheal tube, the other one will try."

"What happens if neither one of them can do it?" asked Howard.

"You cancel the surgery and try again another day. Sometimes a tracheotomy becomes the only way. I'll bet Dr. Kessler has a case or two like that in his bag of horror stories."

"You bet I do. I remember one particularly difficult and bizarre case. The patient was a middle-aged woman who was five feet, three inches tall and weighed about 300 pounds. She had a noticeably short neck and she had a tumor on her vocal cords that had to be removed. Her pre-operative blood gases revealed slightly reduced oxygen. Her PCO_2 was 56.2 – which is very high. She was retaining CO_2 because of her obesity and her frequent attacks of asthma. In fact, she had an asthmatic attack on the very day of her scheduled surgery.

"Surgery should have been cancelled. But, instead, she was anesthetized with drugs. The anesthesiologist – who was working alone, I must add – spent the next 80 minutes attempting to insert a tube into the woman's trachea. He made four such attempts but couldn't get it into her windpipe. During that hour and 20 minutes, the woman's pulse became very rapid – up in the 120s. That's an indication that she wasn't being adequately ventilated.

"Finally, another anesthesiologist was called in to assist. He was able to pass a tube blindly through the nose into the trachea. The throat doctor performing the surgery said he couldn't see the tumor, so he asked the anesthesiologists to reposition the tube. They advanced it a bit and met resistance. That's because the tube was in the right main stem bronchus. They were unable to ventilate the patient because they were only ventilating part of the right lung. So, what should they have done then?"

Dr. Z. and I gave the students an opportunity to field the question. But, when no one replied, she said, "Just pull the tube back up into the trachea and ventilate both lungs with 100% oxygen. That's what they should have done. But what actually happened, Dr. Kessler?"

"They removed the tube completely and tried to ventilate the patient with a mask on the face."

"That was really stupid! Now they'd have to do a tracheotomy really fast!"

"Absolutely," I agreed. "Actually, they did do a tracheotomy, but not before the woman had turned blue and her pulse had become very slow. She went into cardiac arrest and couldn't be resuscitated. Her COD was listed as coronary artery disease because the autopsy showed that one of the woman's coronary arteries was occluded."

"More crap," said Dr. Z. "Her coronary artery may have been occluded, but the cause of death was stupidity, pure and simple."

I TOOK MY STUDENTS to the OR locker rooms where they changed back into street clothes. Nurse Volpe smiled when they handed her their scrubs which they had folded neatly.

"Did you learn anything today?" she asked them.

"We learned how easy it is to kill somebody," Peggy said.

"Good for you, Dear," said Nurse Volpe. "That's really important to remember."

14

FIXING WHAT'S GONE WRONG

━━━

LATE ONE WINTER AFTERNOON in 1972, a doctor friend of mine came to my office and sank down in the armchair beside my desk. "I've got a hell of a problem," he said. I closed the file I'd been reviewing and swiveled around to listen to what he had to say. He was doing some administrative work for an HMO, which ran an emergency room that operated evenings and weekends at a hospital in Queens.

"We're getting our ass sued off," he said.

"What kind of a set up do you have out there?"

"During the day, the ER is staffed by the hospital's regular residents. But at night and on weekends and holidays, it's staffed by a pool of residents from various teaching hospitals around town. They're moonlighting to supplement their regular incomes."

"Can't blame them for doing that," I said. "Who's screwing up? The moonlighters or the hospital house staff?"

"The moonlighters. They work a few hours and then they're gone. They don't have to answer to any superiors, not like the hospital residents who cover the ER on weekdays and who have their own attending physicians to supervise them and help them. The hospital residents know if they screw up, it can affect their promotion in their residency program. Not so the moonlighters."

"What kind of cases are they having trouble with?"

"They're missing a lot of fractures. They can't read X-rays for shit. They're treating patients for sprains and sending them home with broken bones. There's little or no follow-up, so the first indication we have that something's gone wrong is a letter from some lawyer requesting records and X-rays."

"Are these moonlighters training in surgical or non-surgical fields?"

"They're all non-surgical, except for one who's training to be a plastic surgeon."

"Well, right there, that's a big part of your problem," I said. "What you need are more people with a background in trauma. What else are you getting sued for?"

"We're getting sued for delays in diagnosing appendicitis and other causes of acute abdominal pain. I just reviewed a case against us where a man presented to the ER early on a weekend evening with abdominal pain. The moonlighter had the nurses give the patient 100 mg. of Demerol a half hour before actually seeing him. By the time the moonlighter put his hands on the man's belly, the patient was saying he felt much better. And, because his abdomen was soft with minimal tenderness, the moonlighter sent him home with a prescription for narcotics.

"The patient showed up at his own doctor's office two days later with a ruptured appendix and generalized peritonitis. He damn near died. There was severe infection all over his abdominal cavity. Dick, I was taught not to mask symptoms with drugs until I had a diagnosis and a treatment plan."

"You were taught right," I said. "So was I. What you need to do is to get some surgical residents to moonlight. You really need more surgical residents to work along with the internists. They can learn from each other and everybody will benefit, especially the patients."

"That makes sense," my friend said. "Actually, the whole place needs shaking up. I've talked it over with the Powers That Be and they agree. We've hired a new administrator. He's bright and aggressive, and he's looking for a doctor with extensive ER experience who can supervise these doctors. I'd like you to meet him, Dick."

"Hold on, old buddy! I work here full time. I don't think the V.A. wants its full-time people moonlighting."

"This wouldn't interfere with your schedule here. You'd only be on call three or four nights a month. And only one weekend a month. Strictly part-time work. We could really use you because you've had a lot of ER experience."

"But not recently," I told him.

"Even so, it seems to me you're the right kind of guy for the job. How about meeting me there some night? I could make sure the new administrator would be there. You could size him up, take a look around the ER, meet some of the nurses and see what you think. The nursing staff's top-notch, by the way. Very competent and that's a big plus."

The problem in Queens intrigued me. I had to admit that I did have enough experience to at least diagnose what was ailing the troubled ER, even if I couldn't cure it. I had trained at the Washington Hospital Center in the District of Columbia. At the time, it was the fifth busiest emergency room in the country. Fifty percent of all the ambulance calls in the District came to our ER and it was a madhouse on the weekends. I doubted that weekends at the emergency room in Queens could be any more hectic.

I drove out to Queens after work one evening, met with the nursing staff, looked over the facility and sat down with the new administrator. I told him the ER looked fine to me and that the nurses seemed to be terrific. We agreed that the moonlighting residents were the cause of the ER's evening and weekend problem. I told him how I thought I could fix it. He offered me the job and I took it.

HERE'S WHAT WE DID. We started off by hiring more residents with a surgical background. Whenever possible, we arranged to have a resident surgeon and a resident internist work together to provide the broadest possible coverage for the wide variety of medical problems seen in an ER.

I took charge of the residents' work schedule and set it up so that I would have the chance to work side-by-side at least once with each of the doctors from our pool. That allowed me to observe each doctor's work on an individual basis and make sure they understood the new procedures we were putting in place.

"From now on," I told them, "it won't be enough to tell trauma patients that the X-rays taken in the ER don't show any broken bones or fractures. Before you send any trauma patients home, make sure you tell them that the X-ray pictures will be reviewed by a radiologist as soon as possible. Tell them that the radiologist is a specialist and if he sees something you haven't seen, the hospital will call immediately and refer them to an orthopedic surgeon."

I couldn't be at the ER all the time, so I set up an informal X-ray review procedure. Whenever a fracture was missed by an ER doctor or a radiologist, the film was to be placed in a file that I could look over whenever I showed up. I had a highly effective tool I used for these reviews: a big orange grease pencil. Every ER doctor who missed a fracture would be given the X-rays to look at again. It would be impossible to miss the large orange arrow I had drawn which pointed directly at the fracture line. Radiologists who missed a fracture got special treatment. Along with the memo I sent them requesting a corrected X-ray report, I enclosed the original X-ray picture with an even larger arrow pointing to the broken bone.

One radiologist, noted for his mammography skills, seemed to find bones harder to deal with than breasts. He missed several gross fractures. When I sent his X-rays back to him, the arrows I drew were huge. He got the message and, within a short time, so did all the other doctors in the ER. That pretty much took care of the missed fractures problem.

Misdiagnosed bellyaches were also high on my agenda. Hundreds of patients came to the Queens emergency room with abdominal pain. To prevent mistakes, I made it standard emergency room policy that no patient with abdominal pain would be given narcotics, sedatives, tranquilizers or antibiotics until a reasonable diagnosis had been made and the appropriate consultants – surgeons and/or gastroenterologists – had seen the patient and established a treatment plan.

If the patient's abdominal pain was extremely severe, we would permit a small amount of narcotic to be given – provided its effect was evaluated by the examining doctor who had ordered the drug. But under no circumstances would we permit a narcotic to be given to a patient by a doctor who was about to go off duty. We also made it a rule that no patient with undiagnosed abdominal pain would be sent home with a prescription for narcotics, sedatives or antibiotics before a proper diagnosis had been made. That effectively put an end to an egregious practice that had been the cause of so many lawsuits.

I SPENT FIVE YEARS at the ER in Queens. During my tenure, the night and weekend ER staff handled approximately 125,000 patient visits. We were never sued during those five years. Nor was a single chart ever requested by a law firm for review. Looking back, I can see that what I had accomplished was not rocket science. It was the direct result of my own medical training, just a simple matter of sizing up a problem and doing something about it. Diagnose and treat: that's what doctors are trained to do.

A SUDDEN CRY FOR HELP

I WASN'T EXPECTING ANYTHING unusual when I arrived at the Queens emergency room early on a quiet Saturday morning. During the past several months that I'd been supervising the ER night and weekend staff and its procedures, everything had been running smoothly enough. I anticipated nothing more than another normal Saturday in an urban emergency room: some lacerations, bumps and bruises, abrasions and fractures, and a few cases of trauma.

Before doing anything else, I went to my desk and reviewed the X-rays of a couple of fractures that had been missed since my last visit to the hospital. One fracture was overlooked by a staff radiologist and the other by a moonlighting resident. The moonlighting resident, who was an internist, had failed to recognize a small fracture in a finger. The patient, I saw from the records, had already been notified of the break and been referred to his primary care physician for splinting.

Not too bad, I thought. Things were getting better on the weekends since I had instituted some reforms. But the main trouble with the unexpected is that you don't see it coming.

When the moonlighting resident showed up for work in the emergency room that morning, I sat him down and reviewed the X-ray of the fractured finger and gave him some tips on how to avoid making that kind of mistake in the future.

The other X-ray on my desk showed an enormous spiral fracture of the humeral shaft. That arm-bone fracture had been overlooked by the Chief of Radiology, of all people. I drew a large red arrow on the film pointing to the break.

There was a staff radiologist on duty that day and I asked him to drop by my office. When I showed him the film of the spiral fracture and told him that I wanted a revised X-ray report, he was appalled that his boss had failed to recognize a broken arm.

"Yeah," I said. "He's top-notch in his field, but he should stick to mammography."

"You're right, Dr. Kessler, but I can't go asking the chief radiologist for a revised report. He's my boss, after all. I'm just one of the hired help and not one of his favorites, either."

"Okay, okay," I said. "Calm down. I won't get you involved. Getting his attention is all I'm after. I'll put the film on your boss's desk myself, along with a note requesting a revised report. Signed by me, not you." The radiologist thanked me and relaxed.

At that very moment, a woman in the emergency room began screaming. Her shrieks brought us to our feet. "My God!" said the radiologist. "She's *really* in pain!"

We raced to the emergency room. The woman kept screaming. We got to the ER and the moonlighting resident grabbed my arm.

"Thank God, you're here! I don't know what to do for her!"

"Just tell me what's been happening."

"She came in this morning, right after I left your office. Stomach ache, diarrhea. I examined her abdomen. It seemed okay. About a half hour ago, she started complaining about abdominal pain. Then, just now, it suddenly got worse – just like that!."

The woman was still screaming.

"Quick," I said. "What do you know about her?"

"No vomiting. Looks perfectly healthy. Abdomen soft. Not tender. No guarding."

"How old ?"

"About 40."

"Okay, let me take a look." I pulled back the cubicle curtain. The woman saw me and cried out.

"I can't stand it! Oh, my God! Give me something! I've never hurt this bad before!"

"Have you ever had surgery?"

"No!" she gasped. "I've had three babies! This is worse!"

She was writhing in agony, clutching her belly, rolling from side to side. She couldn't find a position that wasn't painful. I put my hands on her abdomen. It wasn't tender. Her bowel sounds were very active.

"Please!" she sobbed, "please give me something!"

"The nurse will give you morphine. That should give you some relief."

"Oh, thank you! Thank you, Doctor!"

I told the ER nurse to give the woman just enough to take the edge off her pain, but not enough to mask her symptoms. Then I took the young medical resident and the staff radiologist out into the corridor.

"I thought at first she might be faking it to get some narcotics," said the resident.

"I see why you might think that, but you can't fake that level of distress. I've seen a few cases where the patient's abdominal pain was way out of proportion to the physical findings."

"So you know what's wrong with her?"

"Maybe," I said. "I hope I'm wrong, but I think she may have intestinal ischemia. That's an acute mesenteric infarction due to occlusion of the arteries in her bowel. If I'm right, something happened to clog or narrow one of her arteries and reduced the supply of blood in her gut. If the tissues in her bowels don't get enough blood, they start to die."

"But her belly is soft," said the resident.

"Yeah, it is. But during the initial ischemic phase, after the occlusion has occurred, the abdomen is always soft. By the time the abdomen becomes tender with guarding, it may be too late. By that time, the bowel is usually dead. We need to get a white blood count on her."

"I drew some blood already," he said. "We should have the test results pretty soon."

"Good. Then I want you to call the chief surgical resident and tell him to get his ass down here stat." While he was doing that,

I turned to the other young doctor, the staff radiologist. "We're going to need an emergency arteriogram of her abdominal vessels."

"I'll get that started," he said. "I'll handle it myself."

Before he could leave, a lab technician rushed in with the blood test results. The woman's white count was 15,400 with a left shift.

"Dammit," I said. I grabbed the young radiologist by the arm. "Wait one minute. Before we do anything else, let's get a plain X-ray of her abdomen to look for a bowel obstruction or a volvulus. That's a twisted bowel, as you probably know."

"I do," he said. "Could that be her problem?"

"I doubt it, but I'd like to rule it out, if we can. That blood count means her bowel is becoming compromised. Pretty soon her belly may become tender. Nurse, has the woman had any diarrhea?"

"Yes," said the ER nurse. "She passed some diarrhea a little while ago. It was bloody."

"Well," I told the medical resident, "that means she's beginning to slough the lining of some of the bowel. It seems to me that this is a classic presentation of acute intestinal ischemia. Where the hell is that surgical resident?"

"He's on his way," said the ER nurse.

"Okay, then let's start another IV and have four units of blood typed and cross-matched."

The morphine was kicking in and the woman had stopped screaming. She was moaning now. I looked behind the curtains and saw that she had raised herself up on her hands and knees and was rocking back and forth on top of the gurney, trying to get comfortable – without success. It took three of us to get her to lay flat so that we could start another IV and place a catheter into her bladder to monitor her urine output.

The chief surgical resident arrived, out of breath. He'd already alerted his surgical team and his attending physician to stand by. He'd found a vascular radiologist to do the woman's emergency arteriogram.

The surgical resident and his team wasted no time prepping the woman for surgery and her operation began just about two hours after she had checked herself into the emergency room.

THERE WAS NOTHING ELSE those of us in the ER could do for the womn, so we got back to work on the few sick and injured people who had begun to trickle in. At one point, a junior surgical resident in scrubs came to the ER to tell us what the arteriogram had shown the surgeons.

"The woman's superior mesenteric artery was occluded," he said, "just beyond its origin from the aorta. And two other arteries were occluded as well. I'll try to keep you posted about the surgery. But it doesn't look good."

"I wish I'd been wrong," I said to my moonlighting resident. "But it looks like my diagnosis was correct."

"I guess so," he said. "I've never seen anything like this."

"It's not common. Most physicians fail to recognize it – or even consider the diagnosis of intestinal ischemia. That's because the physical exam of the abdomen leads them to assume that everything is normal.

"The acute form, like this patient has, strikes suddenly like a bolt of lightening. The key to an early diagnosis is the severity of the pain. It's way out of proportion to anything you might expect, given what you've found in a physical exam.

"The usual cause is a sudden occlusion of the superior mesenteric artery by a clot coming from the heart or from thrombosis – a clotting of the artery that's been slowly occluded by arteriosclerosis."

"But isn't this woman a little young for hardening of the arteries?"

"It can happen to anyone, even a 30-year-old," I told him. "And there are other causes, like clotting in the veins. But no matter what the age or whatever the cause, the patient needs urgent surgery to remove clots or repair a narrowed artery and any dead bowel that has to be resected. You have to act fast."

"And there's no warning?"

"Well," I said, "there is if you've been observing the patient over time and you're able to read the signs. The chronic form of ischemic bowel disease occurs slowly over a period of months or years from progressive occlusion of the intestinal arteries. In chronic cases, patients complain of abdominal pain and often diarrhea soon after eating.

"Gradually, over time, the frequency and severity of their pain increases. Each episode of pain can last up to three hours and their diarrhea may be bloody. As the pain increases in severity, the patient becomes afraid to eat and begins to lose weight.

"So, as a physician, you should be aware that this triad of abdominal pain, diarrhea after eating and weight loss is the classic presentation of chronic intestinal ischemia. The trick is to diagnose the patients' problem with arteriography before they develop the acute phase – what you saw today. It comes on fast and it's often fatal."

"So I guess she's in big trouble up in the OR, isn't she?"

"Yes, she is."

"Have you operated on patients like her?"

"Yeah, that's how I know about all this. There were three or four cases where I was able to resect short segments of dead bowel or restore the circulation in the superior mesenteric artery with a bypass. And I assisted a vascular surgeon in two cases of chronic intestinal ischemia. We did a by-pass graft from the aorta to the superior mesenteric artery.

"But there were at least two dozen cases where all you could do was open them up, look inside, see that there was nothing you could do because most of the bowel was dead, and just close them up. In those cases, I'm sorry to say, the patients experienced a very painful death."

"It seems like a hopeless disease."

"It has a high mortality rate, that's for sure. But some of the bad results are due to doctor delay. Quite often the doctor doesn't think of intestinal ischemia. Or procrastinates before calling a surgeon or getting an arteriogram. Sometimes there's a delay because the doctor has masked the symptoms with large quantities of narcotics. As you've now seen, these patients are gravely ill and they need aggressive supportive measures such as adequate IV fluid therapy."

"I wonder how she's doing up there," the young resident said.

"We'll find out soon enough," I told him. "No news is good news."

THROUGHOUT THE MORNING, whenever there was a break in the ER patient load, the young medical resident and I continued our discussion. He was curious to learn as much as he could about intestinal ischemia and I was more than happy to pass on what I had learned the hard way.

"Sometimes," I told him during one of our breaks, "a physician's error can deprive a patient of a chance for recovery. Just last week, I reviewed a case for a law firm. It's a good example of what we've been talking about. A 51-year-old man went to an ER with sudden, severe abdominal pain and blood in his stool. It was, by the way, Christmas Eve. That's a bad day to get sick.

"He was given narcotics for pain six times that day. Initially, his abdominal exam was normal. By the next day, his abdomen had become tender and distended with a very elevated white blood count indicating that the bowel was becoming gangrenous. He was given narcotics *eight* times that day for the pain. A surgical consult was requested.

"By that evening, the man's blood pressure began to drop; his pulse and respirations went up. By the next morning, he was in a state of severe shock with acute kidney failure because he had only received one quart of IV fluids in eleven hours. He needed two or three times that amount because he weighed about 300 pounds. The pH of the blood was 7.26 and the bicarbonate was 12.9 . . . ."

"Wow! That's *severe* acidosis!" said the resident. "Could dead bowel do that?"

"Absolutely. The surgical consult saw the man for the first time around 7:00 a.m. The consult request, remember, had been made the evening before."

"That's awful."

"Yeah, but remember all this took place on Christmas Day and Christmas Night. During his short hospital stay, ten sets of doctors' orders were entered in the medical record. Six of those were telephone orders. The old HRCS – Holiday Remote Control Syndrome."

"Did they ever operate on this man?"

"Sure, finally. But he was in a state of septic and hypovolemic shock. All but 35 centimeters of small bowel was dead. The right half of the large bowel was gangrenous and had to be removed as well. Now, you can survive with only 35 centimeters of small bowel. But this patient died of shock in the recovery room."

"Do you think he could have survived if they'd operated on Day One?"

"Of course! And it's most probable that a lot more bowel could have been saved if the surgery had been done sooner."

"Are you willing to testify against the doctors?"

"I am. It really pisses me off when doctors don't do the things they're trained to do. But I expect they'll settle out of court, so I won't have to testify."

"Does that sort of delay happen very often? I'd hate to think so."

"It happens often enough. Too often, I'm afraid. I had another case almost identical to the one I just told you about. A 38-year-old obese man went to the ER with severe abdominal pain and bloody diarrhea. The same thing happened to him: multiple doses of strong narcotics, procrastination, inadequate intravenous therapy leading to dehydration – and lots of telephone orders.

"Now, get this! A gastroenterologist and a surgeon both considered intestinal ischemia as a possible cause of the man's symptoms, but they didn't investigate that possibility. The man died of dead bowel before they could do surgery."

"Wow! Thirty-eight years old! That's young!"

"It is," I said. "But here's the point to remember. If you even *consider* the possibility of intestinal ischemia, you have to act quickly. Get X-rays of the intestinal arteries so that if your patient needs surgery, it can be done before it's too late. Take action right away. Not later, not tomorrow, but now. Just like you did today."

"But what *about* patients with chronic intestinal ischemia?" the young resident wanted to know. "How do they do?"

"Much, much better," I answered. "That's providing they're diagnosed before they progress to the acute catastrophic stage. If they're operated on by a vascular surgeon while the bowel is still viable, their survival rate is better than 95%.

"I ran across an interesting physical finding about patients with chronic intestinal ischemia. As the artery or arteries to the bowel slowly become occluded, a bruit can be heard when you place a stethoscope on the abdomen. A bruit, as you probably know, is the *whooshing* sound created by fluid being forced through a narrowed pipe. As long as the bruit can be heard, the artery remains open, albeit narrowed. When the sound of the bruit disappears, you know that the blood supply to the organ beyond the plugged artery is almost completely eliminated. And the shit is about to hit the fan."

"Have you seen cases where the disappearance of a bruit was followed by acute ischemia and dead gut?"

"I've reviewed three cases for law firms where the patients had the classic triad: abdominal pain and diarrhea after eating. They had weight losses of 30-to-70 pounds over periods ranging from six months to three years. Two of the patients had an abdominal bruit, which eventually disappeared, followed very shortly by an acute episode of intestinal ischemia with dead gut that required emergency surgery. Both of them died.

"The third patient was eventually studied with an arteriogram and underwent elective by-pass of the superior mesenteric artery. But he was allowed to become severely dehydrated following surgery. That resulted in gangrene of the bowel. So he died, too."

"Did you testify in those cases?"

"No, they all settled. One case – the case of a 40-year-old woman who had been having classic symptoms and a bruit for over a year – was settled for over $2.5 million. In another, the settlement was very small because the doctor didn't have any malpractice insurance."

"Maybe," said the young resident, "I'll be better off if I don't get malpractice insurance."

"Not a good idea," I said. "That's what doctors call 'going bare.' If you decide to do that, make sure you put all your assets in your wife's name. Otherwise, the patient you screw up can take your house, your car, most of your money and your dog. But you'd better keep your wife happy. If you get divorced, your spouse walks away with it all."

"Maybe I'll just stay single," he said. "But seriously, Dr. Kessler, I don't intend to get sued for malpractice – at least, not for missing a diagnosis of intestinal ischemia and delaying treatment. I'm not going to forget what I learned today."

AS IT TURNED OUT, the young moonlighting resident had one more thing to learn. Shortly after we had sent out for Chinese food, the junior surgical resident from the OR came looking for us.

"It was open and close," he reported. "The woman's bowel was dead from the duodenum to the mid-transverse colon. Nothing could be done. We'll keep her heavily sedated with morphine and she'll be dead by tomorrow, probably. Depressing as hell, isn't it? But we didn't waste any time, thanks to you guys."

With that, he left.

My medical resident sat staring straight ahead, saying nothing. "You did everything you could," I told him.

But that didn't make him feel any better. Me, neither.

16

SHOCK CAN KILL

A LETTER FROM A LAW FIRM I'd been expecting showed up in the mail a few hours before I was scheduled to meet with my third-year medical students to discuss "Shock." Some months before, I had been asked to give an opinion in a small town malpractice case and the lawyers were informing me that their lawsuit had been settled successfully.

Here, I thought, was something I could present to my students one day soon. The case involved a 72-year-old woman who was three days post-op from a colon resection for cancer and a liver biopsy. She was pale, weak and unresponsive. Her abdomen was distended and the hemoglobin numbers had been slowly drifting downward. Her blood pressure was falling and her pulse and respiratory rates were going up. Her urine output was in decline. A surgeon saw her early that Sunday morning. He ordered some blood tests to be done that evening and wrote a bizarre order to get her out of bed. He never saw her again.

Soon thereafter, she was seen by a family practitioner who ordered blood to be transfused as soon as it was available. He also wrote a totally inappropriate order, this one for a psychiatric consult for "post-operative depression." He never saw her again, either.

When I first reviewed the medical records, it was clear to me that the woman had been in shock. She had not needed a psych consult. What she had needed was a doctor at her bedside who would stay with her until the shock was treated successfully with blood transfusions. And, if needed, surgical exploration of her abdomen. Unfortunately for her, this was a small non-teaching hospital that did not have interns or residents.

For the rest of the day, the two doctors were notified repeatedly by the nurses and nursing supervisor about the woman's deteriorating condition. Her blood pressure dropped to 60/48. Her pulse shot up to 133 per minute and her respirations were extremely rapid at 32 per minute. The doctors were difficult to locate and both opted to manage the case by telephone despite being told that, during the entire day shift, the woman's urine output was 60 cc when it should have been 400 to 500 cc.

The first blood transfusion had been ordered at 10:30 a.m., but it was not started until 1:45 p.m. The second unit of blood was given to her at 4:15 p.m. That transfusion took almost three hours when it should have taken about 15 minutes. By 10:15 p.m., the woman's family was demanding that a doctor be in attendance. At 10:30 p.m., the woman was dead.

An autopsy was performed. Four quarts of clots and bloody fluid were found in the woman's abdomen. In all likelihood, this came from the site of her liver biopsy and could have been very easily controlled by early exploration of her abdomen. The family sued the doctors and the hospital.

The first expert witness, hired on behalf of the family doctor, stated that the doctor "practiced within the acceptable standards of care for a family physician and did not contribute to the death" of this patient. God help us all, I thought as I read the transcript, if this is the acceptable standard.

The expert witness for the surgeon tried to shift blame onto the nurses for not keeping the surgeon apprised of the day's events. But the record showed that the nurses had tried hard to locate the surgeon, without success. The surgeon's expert witness also attempted to shift blame onto the family physician by pointing out that he should have transferred the patient to an ICU and followed this up by going to see the patient – rather than playing in a softball game from 4:00 to 6:00 p.m.

I had found this case extremely aggravating to review, so much so that I concluded my expert report with "the management of this case . . . was very deficient and falls far below the standards we expect of medical school graduates who deal with family practice, internal medicine, surgery or gastroenterology. The departures that occurred in this case are so appalling that they are virtually indefensible and should be reported to the State Medical Society for review."

Nowadays I would probably add: "This is not one of those damn frivolous cases that irresponsible politicians and lobbyists keep talking about. Nothing would change their tune quicker than to have their mother or wife or daughter fall victim to a similar medical atrocity."

Well, I thought, I would certainly express that sentiment to my third-year medical students when I presented this case to them. Hopefully, it would encourage them to maintain their youthful enthusiasm to "do no harm" throughout their careers. But it would have to wait for another day. I already had some other shocking stories about "Shock."

WHILE STUDENTS ENTERED the 10th Floor conference room. I listed the four categories of shock on the blackboard: *Cardiogenic, Hypovolemic, Neurogenic* and *Septic.* As soon as all the young men and women were seated at the conference table with pens and note pads at the ready, I began a brief lecture.

"Shock is a clinical syndrome caused by a decrease in the supply of oxygen and nutrients to the various tissues or cells throughout the body. This can result from several causes." I pointed to the first item on the blackboard. "If the heart is damaged and is not pumping to capacity after a heart attack, there will be a reduced blood supply to the tissues resulting in a state called cardiogenic shock.

"If the volume of blood or water in our blood vessels is reduced by hemorrhage or dehydration," I continued, pointing to the second item on the blackboard, "the supply of oxygen and other nutrients to the cells may be reduced sufficiently to cause hypovolemic shock.

"Failure of the nervous system that controls the heart and tone of blood vessels can lead to a condition called neurogenic shock," I said. "That's Number Three." I waited while they finished scribbling in their notebooks before going on.

"Finally, bacteria causing infections can sometime produce toxins that interfere with cellular function and prevent uptake of oxygen and nutrients by the cells. This can lead to septic shock.

"The basic approach to the treatment of shock from any cause is for the doctor to recognize that shock exists or is about to occur and that the treatment must be instigated quickly to restore tissue perfusion before the patient's condition deteriorates beyond the point of no return. Once a state of severe shock exists, there is precious little time available to initiate treatment and prevent irreversible cell damage and death."

The students seemed only mildly interested, so I raised my voice. "There's no room for procrastination! Once informed of the signs and symptoms that suggest that shock exists – or is about to develop – you must ACT NOW! Do not hang up the phone, go back to sleep or take off for the golf course!" That woke them up.

"Now," I said, "what are some of the signs and symptoms of shock?" I put the question to the entire group. "You name them and I'll list them on the blackboard. Come on, let's hear them!"

"A drop in blood pressure and rapid pulse."

"A drop in urine output."

"What else?" I demanded.

"Rapid respiration," a young woman said.

"Absolutely. Why is that?"

"The patient is becoming acidotic from poor tissue perfusion and is trying to blow off CO_2 through the lungs."

"Sure, what else?"

"The skin becomes cold, pale and clammy."

"Very good," I told her. "I can see you've been reading. But the skin isn't always cold. In septic shock, the skin is initially warm. Septic shock patients usually have a high fever and other evidence of infection. If the shock is due to hemorrhage, the hemoglobin and hematocrit in the blood begin to fall. However, the severity of the bleeding is usually underestimated because the fall in the hemoglobin and hematocrit occurs so slowly."

I told the students that I had decided to focus that day's conference on hypovolemic and septic shock, and to give them a couple of cases I thought might get them thinking about what kind of physicians they wanted to be.

"Let's play Doctor," I said. "It's Saturday night in a medium-sized city. You're on duty in your hospital's emergency room. You've all got your degrees. You're all doing well as interns.

"Shortly before midnight, somewhere out in the city, there's a street fight. Someone calls 911. A 17-year-old youth has been stabbed. An ambulance delivers him to your emergency room at 12:15 a.m. That's 25 minutes since he was stabbed. The EMTs wheel him in on a stretcher. He's got an IV running into his left arm.

"You check him over fast. His blood pressure is 100/30, his pulse 120 and his respirations are 30 per minute. You see a three-centimeter laceration in the front of his left upper chest and a three-centimeter laceration in his right flank in the area of his kidney.

"You check his abdomen. It's rigid, but not tender. His blood pressure starts falling. It drops to 80/30. His pulse rate goes up to 140. He's alert, but one of the nurses tells you he's acting 'shocky.' What do you do?"

All the students' hands shot up in the air.

"Get another IV running in the other arm," said the first one I called on.

"How big a catheter?" I asked him.

"Big, big! Maybe a Number 14."

"Speed up the IVs!" urged another student.

"Get a blood sample for type and cross match it for transfusion," a young woman said in a calm voice.

"How many units of blood do you want?" I asked her.

"Two units."

"No, not enough. Don't ever get caught short without enough blood in emergency trauma cases."

"How about six to eight units?" another student said.

"That's more like it. What else do you people want to do?"

The answers came thick and fast. Somehow I managed to write all their answers on the blackboard.

"Measure the hemoglobin and hematocrit."

"Put a catheter into the bladder to measure urine output."

"Get arterial blood gas measurements."

"X-ray the chest."

"Give plasma or a plasma substitute."

I stepped back and scanned the list. "Nice going," I said. "In real life, everything you called for was done in the first 15 minutes. And the youngster's blood pressure rose to 108/44 and his pulse rate came down to 100. What does that suggest to you?"

"His low blood volume was being helped by the IVs," a student answered.

"What were the lab test results?" asked one of the others.

"His hemoglobin was 10.3. Do you think he has bled too much?"

"Oh, yeah," another student replied. "He's lost a lot of blood."

"That's correct," I told him. "And his blood loss is probably even worse than the hemoglobin suggests."

"What did his X-ray show?" another student wanted to know.

"A 30% pneumothorax on the left side – air in the chest with a little bit of fluid. How much blood is a little? Well, it takes at least a pint of blood to show up on a chest X-ray."

"That's not enough to cause this kind of shock," one student stated.

"You're right. Where do you think all the blood has gone?"

"Maybe into his abdomen?"

"Sure," I answered. "He was stabbed in the flank. Maybe the knife penetrated the abdomen or his kidney."

"Is his urine very bloody?"

"No," I said. "That means that his kidney is OK. So we have to look elsewhere. How are you going to test for blood in the belly?"

"Paracentesis."

"What's that?"

He gave me a textbook answer. "It consists of inserting a catheter or needle into the abdomen to aspirate any fluid present."

"Okay." I said. "Then how are you going to deal with his chest injury?"

"Put a chest tube in and suck out air and blood."

"Correct," I said. "Where are you going to put the tube?"

"Anteriorly – under the third or fourth rib, "

"Right," I said. "And that was also done in the first 15 minutes. What do you think came out?"

"Blood and air, right?" said the student.

I nodded.

"What did the paracentesis show?" he asked.

"It wasn't done," I told him. "They sucked out the air and blood through the chest tube, but they didn't do a paracentesis. Don't ask me why, because I don't have any idea. But they certainly should have done it."

Another student broke in to ask, "Do we have the results of the blood gases?"

"Yes, we have that," I answered, "The pH was 7.10, which is very low. The HCO3 was 13, also very low. So what does that tell you?"

"It tells me that this is severe shock causing acidosis," a young woman said. "No doubt about it."

I gave her a nod of approval and continued my presentation.

"Fifteen minutes after the young man was admitted, the ER called a thoracic surgeon. He got all the information I've given you – over the phone. He said that a 30% pneumothorax and such a small amount of blood could not cause shock. He advised the ER to consult the general surgeon who was on call at the hospital. That was done and that surgeon arrived about 30 minutes later. So where has all this youngster's blood gone?"

"Into the abdomen." My student was sticking with his original answer.

"And where else?" I asked, but nobody had that answer.

"The street," I said. "He probably spilled a lot of blood at the scene of the knife fight. The important thing to remember is that the ER nurse had said 'he is shocky' – as she put it – and 'his hemoglobin is very low.' So what do you want to do now?"

"Is the blood ready for transfusion?"

"It should be," I said. "It's been 45 minutes. That's how long it takes to type and cross match blood. But suppose his blood pressure is falling and the blood is not ready yet. What to you do?"

Again, no answer.

"You go with O-Negative blood, if you have it. O-Negative is the universal donor, but it's always in short supply. This patient was O-Positive, the most common type, so they could have used O-Positive without cross match in this sort of emergency. The U.S. Army got through WWII with O-Positive blood.

"Anyway, they took the young fellow to the OR at 2:00 a.m. to explore his abdomen. The anesthesia was started at 2:05 a.m. Do you know how long it should take a surgeon to wash his hands, gown up and drape the patient?" No one ventured a guess, so I told them. "Five to 10 minutes at the most in an emergency like this one where a person may be bleeding to death. In this case, it took the surgeon 35 minutes. Again, don't ask me why. It just did."

"What did they find?" I was asked.

"Nothing. And they wasted a helluva lot of time performing an exploratory operation. They wouldn't have had to perform that exploratory surgery if they had done a paracentesis in the first place. They started out doing things just fine. But then they began dropping the ball. Do you know how long it should take to open and close an abdomen when nothing has been found?"

"About half an hour?"

"That's about right. But this kid was under anesthesia for one hour and 45 minutes and, throughout the procedure, his blood pressure was at shock levels."

"How much blood did they give him?" a student asked.

"Up to this point, he had not received a blood transfusion."

"My God, that's terrible!"

"It sure is," I said. "Now, get this: The medical records show that the reason the exploratory operation took so long was because they screwed around sewing up the lacerations in the flank, chest, ear and wrist. That ate up a lot of time"

"What drugs did they use to help raise his blood pressure?"

"None," I answered. "They didn't give him anything."

I waited until the students stopped making angry noises. "There's more. At the end of the procedure, the surgeon put a large tube into the lower part of the youngster's chest and removed 900 to 1,000 cc of blood. That's a full quart of blood! So what should he have done then?"

"Call the thoracic surgeon," several students said at once.

"He did that," I said, "but not for two hours."

"You've got to be kidding! When the hell *did* the patient get a blood transfusion?"

"He got his first blood transfusion an hour and 10 minutes after the operation. At 5:15 a.m. – five hours after being rolled into the ER."

"That's terrible," one student sighed.

"I agree," I said, "but it gets worse. The thoracic surgeon – the same guy who failed to answer his call to duty at 12:30 a.m. – finally begins chest surgery at 6:45 a.m. That's because the young man had gone into cardiac arrest after the first operation and had to be resuscitated.

"Now he was back on the table for a suture of a laceration of the upper lobe of the left lung and ligation of a branch of the pulmonary artery. He was given a total of seven units of blood – a bit too late, wouldn't you say? Anyway, after this second operation he remained in shock with dilated and fixed pupils. At 4:40 in the afternoon, he was pronounced dead."

"I'll bet the thoracic surgeon felt like a damn fool," a student exclaimed.

"You would think so," I said. "Maybe he learned to get the hell out of bed when the situation demands it. But don't forget that the general surgeon also dropped the ball."

"Did the case end up in court?" a young woman asked. I told her it had gone to trial, but that the defense was able to convince the jury that the youngster's case was hopeless from the start, even before he arrived in the ER.

"But here's something that you should never forget," I told the young men and women sitting around the conference table. "When someone is bleeding to death, you give them *blood!* And lots of it!"

I WAITED WHILE A VOLUNTEER erased my notes from the blackboard – that's one of the perks of being a teacher – and then started in on the next case.

One Saturday afternoon in a small middle-American town, a 50-year-old man suffered abdominal trauma on his job in a lumberyard. A piece of wood flew off a buzz saw he was working with and struck him hard just above the pubis.

He was in such pain that his boss rushed him to the emergency room of the local hospital. According to the medical record, he arrived in the ER at 3:15 p.m. He had an abrasion across the skin of his lower abdomen. The area where his skin was scraped was very tender. There was severe (4+) guarding of the muscles in that region of his abdomen.

"In fact," I said, "the man's abdomen was so hard, the doctor couldn't push it in to test for rebound tenderness. The man's pulse was 60, his respirations 24 per minute and his blood pressure was 114/70. His bowel sounds were reduced. There was nothing significant in his past medical history except for an appendectomy 30 years before.

"So what do you guys want to do with this man? Give him some Percoset and send him home, maybe?"

"Oh, no," a student replied. "He's got to be admitted and observed."

"Why?" I challenged him. "He probably just has a bad bruise of the muscles and they're bound to be very tender for at least a week. He'll need a little something for the discomfort."

"But he may have something serious going on," said the student, standing his ground. "It's too early to tell."

"Oh, yeah?" I said. "Something serious? Like what?"

"Maybe a ruptured bladder."

"OK, that's worth considering." I went to the blackboard and wrote *Differential Diagnosis* at the top and started making a list.

"We know he has a bad bruise." I wrote *Bad Bruise* on the blackboard. "Could he have a ruptured bladder? Maybe. So we'll make that *Ruptured Bladder* Number 2. What else could have been injured?" I asked a timid student.

"How about a fractured pelvis?"

"Good!" I said. "That's a distinct possibility and we'll make *Fractured Pelvis* our Number 3. What else?"

"Maybe he's bleeding internally?" another student said.

"Bleeding from where?"

"Maybe some vessels in the abdomen?"

"What vessels?"

"What about the aorta?"

"No way," I said. "If it was his aorta, he would have been DOA – dead on arrival."

"Well, then, how about the vena cava and iliac veins?"

"That's better," I said. "Blunt trauma to the pelvis or the abdomen can cause bleeding behind the peritoneum. It's called 'retroperitoneal hematoma.' The bleeding is usually of venous origin and it can occur slowly. And we'll make *Retroperitoneal Hematoma* 4-A on our list. But what else could be bleeding?"

I waited about 10 seconds for them to come up with an answer, but they couldn't. So I explained that this kind of injury could also tear a blood vessel going to the bowel and I listed *Mesenteric Vessels* as 4-B.

"Could his bowel itself be ruptured?" a student asked.

"Sure," I said. "Absolutely. Number 5 is *Rupture of the Bowel.* But that's less likely because the bowel is very mobile. A blunt force like this one would push the bowel aside. It would be more likely to injure fixed structures like the bladder or major blood vessels. But it's possible."

I put the chalk back in its tray and went back to the conference table. "So, what are we going to do with this guy?"

"Admit him to the hospital and observe him," someone said.

"That's right. And his doctor did that. Are you going to feed the patient?"

"No, you want him to have an empty stomach if surgery is an option."

"That's right again. And his doctor did not feed him."

"How about an IV for fluids?" another student asked.

"Sure, that's a good idea. And his doctor did that. Are you going to give the injured man anything for pain?"

"No," one of the young women responded. "We don't want to relieve his pain until we're sure about what's happening with him. Strong medicine could mask his symptoms."

"Well, maybe you could just give the poor man a little something so that he could get some sleep?"

"No," she said quickly. "And for the same reason."

"Very good," I said. "You don't want to mask his symptoms and the records show that his doctor did not give him any drugs. Now, let me ask you how frequently you want the nurses to check his vitals – his temperature, pulse and blood pressure?"

"Every 15 to 30 minutes."

"You're right," I said. "But the man's doctor ordered his vital signs to be checked once every four hours."

"Every four hours? That's not enough, is it?"

"I'll say it isn't. This doctor is beginning to deviate from good practice. Now, let's say you are the doctor. How often would you want to examine this patient?"

"Every two hours?" a young woman ventured and the others agreed with her.

"Every two hours at the very least," I said. "Doctors have to stay on top of trauma cases. If vital signs become abnormal, you may have to stay with the patient continually. I should mention that this doctor didn't see this patient again for 11 hours."

Several of the students shook their heads in disbelief.

"But let's say that, unlike this doctor, you have written your basic orders correctly. The man's vitals are to be checked frequently, at least every two hours or less. What diagnostic tests would you want done now so that you can evaluate your differential diagnoses list? You know the man has a contusion of the abdominal wall. So how do you evaluate a possible rupture of the bladder?"

"Can he void?" a student asked.

"Yes," I told him.

"What color is his urine?"

"Yellow," I said, "but a microscope has detected red blood cells in the urine."

"Well, then! He probably does have a ruptured bladder!"

"Not likely," I told the class. "In most cases when the bladder is ruptured, the urine is grossly bloody. However, you'd want to put the issue to rest. So what test can be done to rule out a ruptured bladder?"

"A cystogram," someone answered.

"What's that?" I asked.

"You inject a dye into the bladder through a catheter and take X-rays."

"Correct. And that was done in this case. It was normal."

"How about Number 3 on the list?" a young man asked. "The fractured pelvis."

"Yeah," said another student. "Get an X-ray."

"That was done. No fracture. But what about Number 4 up there – Hemorrhage?"

"Do a blood count and then check the hemoglobin and hematocrit."

"That was done, too," I said. "The white count was normal, the hemoglobin was 15 and the hematocrit was 45."

"That's high normal," a student said, "so it doesn't appear that he's bleeding."

"Well, what about Number 5 – Ruptured Bowel?"

All the students had the same answer. "Get flat and upright X-rays of the abdomen!"

"Why do you want an upright X-ray? What are you looking for?"

"Free air in the belly because of a perforated bowel."

"That was done and it was normal. Does that rule out a perforated gut?" The students all said it did.

"You're all wrong," I said. "A normal upright X-ray doesn't rule it out. Not at all. This kind of patient has to be sitting up for 15 to 20 minutes before getting an upright X-ray. That gives any free air enough time to rise up to the diaphragm where it will show up on the X-ray film. Even then, a negative test does not – and I repeat – does not rule out a perforated bowel. Don't ever forget that."

"How about ordering an ultrasound or a CT scan?"

"It wasn't available in that small town hospital," I told him. "But you probably wouldn't need it anyway. What would you be looking for?"

"A dilated bowel. Fluid in the belly, maybe. And, by the way, Dr. Kessler, where was this town?"

"Buffalo Breath, Montana," I said with a straight face. "I'm just kidding. It was just your average small town. Could have been anywhere. But let's get on with the case.

"At 2:30 in the morning, the nurse on duty calls the doctor and tells him that all is not well. He goes to see the patient immediately. The man appears to be sicker. His temperature is 101 degrees, pulse 120 and blood pressure 120/60. His abdomen is distended and very rigid with definite rebound tenderness. His urine output has decreased. And now he has pain in his left shoulder. What do you make of that?"

"It sounds like he has peritonitis," a student said. "What's his white blood count?"

"Slightly elevated," I responded.

"What about the hemoglobin?" another student asked.

"It's 17. Now, what does that mean?"

"It tells me that he's not bleeding and he's probably dehydrated."

"Very good," I said. "But what about the man's shoulder pain?"

"Did the lumber hit him in the shoulder?" a young woman asked.

"No," I told her, "his shoulder wasn't injured in the accident. It moves freely and it's not tender. So what's causing the left shoulder pain?"

Third-year medical students seldom have an answer to this question, so I gave them a hint. "Maybe there's something irritating the undersurface of the diaphragm?"

"Something like pus?" one student said. "Maybe it could be something like pus."

"Or like blood," the others chimed in. "Or like intestinal contents." "Or air?"

"Well, you're all correct," I said. "So what's your diagnosis?"

It took them only a few moments to agree on "perforated bowel with peritonitis."

"How could you test for pus or fluid in the belly?" I asked.

"Would a paracentesis help?"

"Absolutely," I said. "And it's not expensive to just insert a needle into the belly and aspirate up into a syringe. So what do you do now?

The students had a lot of suggestions: Call a surgeon. Increase the IVs. Put a Foley catheter into the bladder to monitor urine output. Pass an NG tube into the stomach and insert a central venous catheter.

"You're all on target," I said. "And all your suggestions were carried out. So when would you call the surgeon?"

"Right away!" a young man said.

"Yes, right now," I replied. "But this doctor waited a full eight hours before calling the surgeon." The students groaned. "The man was finally seen by the surgical consult at ten o'clock in the morning. He was gasping for air. His blood pressure was 98/60, his pulse was 128 and his respirations were now 36. The surgeon concluded that his patient either had a contusion of the bowel or a retroperitoneal hematoma."

"How could he think that? The hemoglobin had gone up instead of down!"

"Beats me," I replied. "Anyhow, he decided to wait and see."

"He must have been an idiot," someone growled.

"Probably not," I said. "But he certainly wasn't thinking clearly that Sunday morning. By 5:30 p.m. – that was 24 hours since the man was admitted – ten and a half quarts of IV fluids had been used to keep his urine output at 2,700 cc. A central venous line had been inserted and the central venous pressure was now zero."

"That means he's losing a lot of fluid into his belly and is hypovolemic!"

"Right on," I said. "By four o'clock in the morning, Monday morning, the man's respirations were 50 and his temperature was 103. Bowel sounds were absent and there was no urine output. He was very distended. His blood pressure was 80/60. The surgeon sees the patient, realizes the man has developed septic shock and decides to operate."

"About time!" a student exclaimed.

"Did the surgeon find out what was perforated?" another asked.

"He found five holes in a short segment of the terminal small bowel which was stuck to the back of the abdomen by adhesions. The piece of wood had crushed this segment of bowel against the spine and it had burst. The surgeon sutured each hole and irrigated the abdomen which was severely infected and full of small bowel contents."

"This infection, Dr. Kessler? Was it under the diaphragm? That would explain the shoulder pain."

"Yes, it was. And, yes, it does explain it," I said.

"Did they use antibiotics or drugs to support the blood pressure?"

"Yes, they did. But to no avail. Nothing was going to be successful without early surgery. By the next day, the man's pulse had gone up to 150 and then dropped to 40. His temperature was 104 and his blood pressure fell to 40/0. That's correct – 40 over zero! His urine output fell to zero. The pupils of his eyes became dilated and that's an indication of brain damage. He died of sepsis the next day."

The students sat in silence for a minute or so. Finally, one of them asked if it had been a wise decision to suture the five holes in the terminal small bowel.

"No, it wasn't," I answered, "The odds of all five of those sutured holes remaining intact were close to zero. Ileostomy and colonic mucous fistula would have been a better choice. That is to say: the surgeon could have resected that short segment and brought the bowel out through the skin. If the man had survived, the continuity of bowel could have been restored several weeks or months later. But then, he didn't survive, did he?"

"Were the doctors sued?"

"Yes, and sued successfully. The jury awarded the family $200,000."

"Is that all? It doesn't seem like much."

"The family was okay with that, I heard, but the lawyer wasn't too happy. He'd invested a lot of his own money to have the case reviewed and presented to the jury. But don't forget that this happened in a small town. I grew up in a small town in upstate New York and I know it's hard for small town people to think in terms of millions like we do here in New York City. But that's not what I want you to remember about this case."

I TOOK A MOMENT to survey the serious, attentive young men and women seated around the conference table. "If you remember anything about this case, remember this," I said. "If you are ever observing a patient with blunt abdominal trauma and any vital signs become abnormal – I mean pulse, blood pressure, temperature, respirations or urine – you should be aware immediately that you're dealing with something really bad.

"If the patient's pain increases or moves to the shoulder, know that you must explore that patient's abdomen even if X-rays, ultrasounds or CT scans are normal. The fact that this small town hospital didn't have expensive, hi-tech, big-city diagnostic tools is irrelevant. They weren't needed. The symptoms were there in plain sight.

"This man's abdomen should have been opened up and explored within 12 hours after he showed up in the ER. If that had been done, he'd probably be alive today."

17

A NICE OLD BLOATED MAN

D ID YOU KNOW THAT some doctors don't have a clue about "bloat? That is to say: they don't know how to manage cases of abdominal distension or bowel obstructions. I became aware of that fact long before I ever started to review medical malpractice cases.

As an intern and as a resident, I had seen the results of the mistakes made by some doctors who treated their patients' symptoms without looking for the cause of their distress. If their patients vomited, they gave them an anti-emetic to stop the nausea and the vomiting. If a patient had a history of constipation, they prescribed laxatives, enemas or suppositories. Did the patient have diarrhea? They'd administer an oral solution to slow down bowel activity. In short, they treated the symptom, not the problem.

One of the most appalling acts of medical stupidity I ever encountered involved bloat. It took place in a nursing home in upper Manhattan. I had gone up there to see a lawyer friend of mine who worked there as nighttime administrator. While we were having dinner, Sol asked me for a favor.

"We have an old man upstairs who's very bloated. I'm really worried about him, Dick."

"Has he seen a doctor?"

"I understand that a proctologist saw him yesterday and gave him something for diarrhea."

"Bloating and diarrhea? To me, that sounds like a bowel obstruction, Sol. I'd be happy to take a look at him, if you want me to." And so, after dinner, we took a slow ride up to the third floor in an ancient, manually operated elevator. The elevator and its operator seemed to be as old and creaky as the building. And so, I was to learn, were some of its medical practices.

"Max is a nice old guy," said Sol. "Sharp as a tack mentally, but his body's failed. He's got advanced Parkinson's and he's basically bedridden. And now, well, you'll see for yourself."

Max gave us a wave and a smile when we entered his room. He was a skinny little man but his belly made him look like he was nine months pregnant. Bloat from gas, I said to myself.

"This is my friend, Dr. Kessler, Max. I asked him to take a look at you."

"So, look," said Max. "I'm not going anywhere. Is this going to cost me?"

"No charge," I said. "Sol bought me dinner."

"I hope it was at a restaurant," said Max. "If you ate here, you're going to need a doctor yourself. So, what do you want me to do?"

"Nothing," I said. "Just lie there and let me poke around."

"Why not?" said Max.

His belly sounded like a drum when I tapped my fingers on it. When I checked his abdomen with my stethoscope, I heard the tinkling sound of gas and fluid. I took Max's chart from the foot of his bed and read through it. I saw that he had been bloated and having diarrhea for over two weeks. I was shocked to read that the proctologist who had seen Max the day before had "*deferred rectal exam because of diarrhea.*"

"So what do you think, Doc?" said Max. "Think you can sell my story to the movies? I'll give you ten percent of the net. Not the gross. I'm old, but I'm not stupid."

"You've got a deal," I said. "But first I'll have to check out your nurse and make sure she's right for the part."

"Go take a look," said Max. "She's just down the hall. I don't know if she can act, but she's got her own costume."

Once outside Max's room, I said to my friend, "For Christ's sake, Sol, the idiot didn't do a rectal exam! Can I borrow your nurse? And some rubber gloves? Somebody's got to do a rectal on this poor guy! And right away, too!"

"You're going to do it, Dick?"

"Who else?" I said. "In the hospital, I can usually find a resident to do it. And the resident can find an intern, who will try to find a medical student. But here and now, it's just you and me and the nurse."

After a short conference in the nurse's office, the three of us returned to Max's bedside. I turned him over on his side and started to perform a rectal examination. I didn't get far. Max's rectum was full of hard stool. I stepped back and shook my head. "Well," I said to Sol and the nurse, "I think I've discovered the problem."

"Are you going to let me in on it?" said Max. "Or is it a secret?"

"Well, Max, it appears to me that you haven't had a bowel movement for a while."

"Seems like forever. I can't remember the last time."

"Yeah," I said. "So what you've got is a fecal impaction and that's caused bowel obstruction."

"You're telling me I'm full of shit," said Max. "Don't worry. You're not the first one to tell me. So, you can do something about it?"

"You bet I can, Max. But it's going to take a little time and it's going to be uncomfortable. But your nurse will give you something to make it a little easier."

"You left out embarrassing," said Max. "Uncomfortable, I can take. But embarrassment? You got something I can take for that?"

"I'm afraid not, Max. I could blindfold Sol and your nurse, but I'm going to need their help to get all that stool out of your rectum. Once that's done, you'll feel a lot better. I'll be as gentle as I can."

Max patted me on the arm. "I know you will, Doctor," he said. "So, go wash your hands. You too, Sol. I wouldn't want to catch something."

I took the nurse out into the hallway and told her what I would need – a rubber sheet, a couple of bedpans and some extra surgical gloves. "I always wear two pairs of gloves when I have to do this sort of thing," I told her. "I learned the hard way that the odor of stool will go right through one glove and permeate the skin of the fingers. It takes several days to get rid of the stink."

Sol and I went to the Men's Room to empty our bladders and wash up. "What I'm going to do," I explained to him, "is probably going to take from one or two hours. Max has a mass of hard stool about the size of a football, I'd guess. It must fill up his entire pelvis. I've got to break up that fecal impaction because that's what blocking his bowels."

"But he's got diarrhea," said Sol.

"That's right," I said. "Liquid stool above the mass is being forced around the hard stool and that's why he has diarrhea. The proctologist who saw him yesterday prescribed medication to stop the diarrhea, but that was just plain stupid. When it comes to severe fecal impaction, medication to stop diarrhea doesn't work. Enemas don't work and suppositories don't work either. The only thing that works is manual removal. And that's us, old buddy."

Sol looked a bit pale. "Just what do you want me to do, Dick?"

"Just keep emptying the bed pans, Sol. Make sure I've always got a clean, empty one in reserve." I dried my hands with a couple of paper towels. "Thank God that proctologist didn't prescribe a laxative," I said. "That could have perforated Max's bowel – and that could have been fatal."

We walked back to Max's room. The nurse had given Max his medication and he seemed to be comfortable and relaxed on the rubber sheet she had spread across his bed. I asked Max how he was feeling.

"Wonderful, simply wonderful," he murmured. "I am closing my eyes and thinking of England."

"That's good, Max. And I'm pulling up a chair, sitting down and putting on two pairs of white gloves just for the occasion. It's okay by me if you drift off. You'll feel better pretty soon." Max made no reply. All I could hear was his steady breathing. Good for him, I thought.

And so I set to work. I had to work slowly and carefully to avoid any injury to the rectum. It took a long time to break up the hard mass so that I could start removing impacted stool piecemeal. Fortunately, I had called my family in New Jersey to tell them I would be late getting home.

By the time I was finished, I had filled two bedpans with stool. But once I had removed about half of the mass, a channel opened and that allowed the passage of large amounts of liquid and gas. Sol was kept busy emptying and cleaning the bedpans. It was a long, difficult and dirty procedure. But, before we were halfway through, we could see Max's abdominal distension disappearing rapidly. When it was over and all of us had washed up, Max held both my hands in his and thanked me.

"I haven't felt this good in months," he said. "Sol, take this wonderful doctor out and buy him a couple of drinks. He should feel as good as I do!"

Sol did just that and the nurse joined us at the bar down the block when her shift ended. "I think we have good reason to celebrate tonight," said Sol. "It's my considered legal opinion that Dick not only helped a sweet old man, he also saved the nursing home from a real nasty lawsuit."

"And it's my considered opinion," said the nurse, "that you two may be suffering from acute celebration syndrome which can sometimes be fatal. I prescribe taxicabs. Take two and call each other in the morning."

18

TERMINAL BLOAT

━━━

I ALWAYS TOLD RESIDENTS that "the sun should never set on a fecal impaction because the hard stool may erode into the bowel wall causing ulcers, bleeding and perforation. And don't forget to use two pairs of gloves. The important thing is that somebody must remove the hardened stool – by hand. Failure to do it is negligence. Wasting time by trying to relieve the impaction with enemas and laxatives may prove fatal."

I learned that when a law firm in New Jersey asked me to review the case of a 15-year-old girl who was admitted to the hospital at 1:30 a.m. with a two week history of chronic constipation, rectal bleeding, weakness plus the inability to urinate for one day. She was pale, thin and emaciated. Her abdomen was distended hard and non-tender. Her blood pressure was 100/60, her pulse 120 and her respirations 24 per minute. Her temperature was normal. Blood and blood clots were coming out of her anus.

Rectal examination revealed a hard, massive fecal impaction filling her rectum. Abdominal X-rays revealed a large amount of stool in the large bowel and rectum. This was causing dilation of the bowel which in turn pushed up against the diaphragm to such an extent that her lung capacity was reduced by 50 percent. Her white blood count was elevated at 17.0 with a left shift. Her hematocrit was low at 22.0.

Over the next three days she was treated with IVs, laxatives and enemas. Her temperature was only slightly elevated, but her pulse remained rapid. Her abdomen became more distended and tender. No one did a manual removal of the stool from the rectum. The enemas and laxatives accomplished nothing.

One night at 10:00 p.m. – almost three days after she had been admitted to the hospital – the girl became severely distended, very pale, confused, cyanotic and extremely short of breath. Her blood pressure began to fall, first to 90/70, then to 80/60 while her abdomen exhibited a board-like rigidity and was tender all over. Her respirations were 30 per minute and shallow.

A house doctor saw her and started another IV, drew blood for tests and for the preparation of blood for transfusion. At this juncture, the girl's hemoglobin was down to 6.2, an indication that she had lost a great deal of blood and was in shock. So the doctor finally tried to vigorously remove the stool from her rectum manually. He removed large amounts of hardened stool and that provided a route for equal amounts of gas to be expelled.

His action came too late. The girl died as she was being transferred to the ICU and she could not be resuscitated.

The house doctor had proved that the fecal impaction could have been manually removed if someone had made the effort. But this should have been done on Day One – not three days later when she had already entered a state of shock.

It is well known that fecal impactions cause rectal bleeding, yet this patient never received a blood transfusion. The final insult was most probably the perforation of distended bowel. However, the actual cause of the terminal event is not certain because no autopsy was performed.

It was my opinion that the hospital staff, intent on using laxatives and enemas instead of manual removal, wasted precious time and probably cost this teenager her life. But the doctors who cared for this patient were successfully defended at trial by very competent lawyers who convinced the jury that the patient had waited too long before seeking medical treatment. There is, I suppose, some merit to that suggestion. At least, the jury thought so.

EVERY TIME A NEW GROUP of third year medical students was assigned to my surgical service, I was required to conduct a conference on intestinal obstruction and this was my afternoon to tell my new students about "The Bloat." Once they were all seated around the conference table, I went to the blackboard and wrote the topic in chalk: *Abdominal Distension.*

"Abdominal distention is an ominous sign," I began, "except when it's caused by pregnancy. If it is due to the accumulation of large amounts of fluid, it means severe liver disease or terminal cancer. But, usually, abdominal distension is caused by the retention of gas within the bowels. When the bowels become blocked – whether by hernia, scar tissue (adhesions), tumor or stool – intestinal contractions are unable to expel the gas or stool beyond the obstruction. The fluid and gas back up. And this leads to vomiting and abdominal distension.

"Now if the obstruction is not relieved, the bowels become more and more distended and may reach a point where the bowel ruptures and spews intestinal contents into the abdominal cavity. This is a disaster! It leads to severe infection and often death.

"The goal of treatment is to relieve the distension before the bowel ruptures. The patient should not be fed. A tube should be passed through the nose into the stomach and connected to a suction machine. The use of drugs alone to stop vomiting is contraindicated in patients with intestinal obstruction."

I wrote *Levin Tube* on the blackboard. "It rhymes with *begin*," I said and turned toward the conference table. "The Levin suction tube is a very useful device to suck out gas and fluid. Many patients with intestinal obstructions will require surgery to alleviate the condition whether it was caused by a tumor or by adhesions – scar tissue.

"The most common cause of gaseous abdominal distension is a *Paralytic Ileus.* This is a condition where the bowel is temporarily paralyzed and unable to push the intestinal contents forward. The gas and fluids in the bowel accumulate, resulting in dilation of the bowel. If it is not relieved, the bowel may become so wide that it can perforate. And that leads to severe infection in the abdomen.

"Abdominal pain, abdominal surgery, bowel manipulation during surgery, abdominal infections, kidney stones, pancreatitis, fractures of the spine – these are all conditions that may cause paralytic ileus. If distension and vomiting occur because of an ileus, the patient should not be fed. And a tube should be inserted into the stomach to prevent further distension of the bowel. Failure to use a Levin tube or feeding a patient who is vomiting can make the ileus worse."

I wrote *Ogilvie's Syndrome* on the blackboard. "Ogilvie's Syndrome is a severe form of ileus that affects the large bowel. This syndrome occurs in elderly bedridden patients who already may be afflicted with a wide variety of illnesses. Patients with liver, kidney, pancreatic and spinal diseases are prone to this complication. Alcoholics and even cardiac patients may develop this unusual form of large bowel distension.

"The distension usually involves the right half of the colon. If it's not relieved, the distended large bowel may rupture and lead to a virulent infection. Rupture of the colon is likely if the beginning portion of the large bowel – the cecum – is allowed to get larger than 10-to-12 centimeters.

"The treatment is passage of a long tube – a colonoscope – up the rectum to suck out the air that is causing the distension. This works 90% of the time and may need to be repeated. If colonoscopy is not successful, then a tube has to be inserted into the cecum for decompression cecostomy."

After these opening remarks, I turned to the blackboard and wrote *Differential Diagnosis*. I could hear the students behind me coming to full attention. The lecture was over.

"The first case we'll discuss today," I said, "is that of a 63-year-old male who was admitted to the hospital on a New Year's Eve."

"That's a bad day to get sick," a student whispered to his neighbor.

"Do you know why?" I asked the Whisperer.

"There's a huge reduction in hospital staff during holidays. Most people are out celebrating."

"That's absolutely true," I said. "But this patient probably had no choice. He showed up on New Year's Eve with a one-week history of abdominal cramps, vomiting, abdominal distension, hiccups, weight loss and failure to have a bowel movement. What's your differential diagnosis?"

"Intestinal obstruction," several students volunteered. I wrote *Intestinal Obstruction* on the blackboard.

"OK, what is the most common cause of intestinal obstruction?"

"Has he ever had abdominal surgery?" asked one of my brighter students.

"Very good," I told her. "No previous surgery. This was a virgin abdomen he presented."

"Then I'd say groin hernia. It's probably the most common cause of a bowel obstruction in a virgin abdomen."

"You're absolutely right. Now let's suppose, hypothetically, that there was a scar on the man's abdomen. What would you then say would be the most common cause of obstruction?"

"Adhesions or scar tissue from the previous surgery now blocking the bowel," she said. "But that's not the case here. Our man has never had surgery."

"Right," I said, picking up the chalk. "So Number One is *Groin Hernia*. Number Two is *Adhesions*. And what's Number Three?"

"Tumor," several students replied at the same time.

"Right again," I said and added *Tumor* to the list. "Now this man was very sick. His BUN – his kidney function test – was 65. Why is that?"

"He's been vomiting and he's very dehydrated."

"Good point. Why is he hiccupping?" Nobody answered so I dropped a hint. "Maybe something is irritating the diaphragm?"

"Oh, yeah!" an eager student said. "He's perforated his bowel."

"Not necessarily. His abdomen is very distended but it's not tender."

"What did the X-ray show?" another student asked.

"The small bowel was very dilated," I told him.

"Can distended bowel or stomach irritate the diaphragm?" asked a student who seldom spoke up in class.

"Sure it can. Absolutely."

"Did he have a hernia, Dr. Kessler?"

"Yes, he did. There was a solitary firm lump in the left groin. Now that we know that, how are we going to manage this case?"

"Hydrate him with IVs," a student replied, "and fix the hernia."

"You got it. That was an easy case wasn't it? Well, not as it turned out. The man was started on IVs alright, but unfortunately he was observed without benefit of a surgical consult."

A freckle-faced redhead interrupted. "May I ask where the hell this happened?"

"At a world famous teaching hospital in Boston, Sean. Anyhow, on the man's third hospital day, a CT scan showed massive distension of the stomach and the small bowel with a loop of small bowel within a left inguinal hernia.

"You'd think they would have operated on him right then, but they didn't. His doctors continued to observe him without a surgical consult. And on the sixth day, he aspirated vomitus and developed pneumonia."

"Didn't they have a nasogastric tube in place?"

"No, not until after he had aspirated large quantities of foul, fecal-smelling liquid which came from his stomach. The very next day, still without the benefit of a surgical consult, he developed septic shock and died."

"That's appalling," said the redhead.

"You bet it is. The autopsy showed that the man's bowel had perforated eight inches above the hernia. Two-and-a-half quarts of foul, purulent fecal material were found in his abdominal cavity."

I let that sink in and then told the students, "Always remember whenever you see a patient with a bloated abdomen and a lump in the groin, you're dealing with an obstructing hernia – until proven otherwise."

I WHEELED A PORTABLE X-ray viewing box to the table. "Our next case is that of a 38-year-old woman who was admitted to the hospital with a one-day history of abdominal pain associated with constipation and the vomiting of fecal smelling fluid. What other information do you want for a differential diagnosis?"

"What did an X-ray of the abdomen show?"

I removed several X-rays from a large folder and placed two of them on the view box. "What do you see?" I asked.

"Dilated loops of bowel with fluid levels."

"Correct. And note the stepladder effect of the fluid levels. That's typical of a mechanical obstruction. Also, she had surgery on an ovary several years before. Knowing that, what's Number One on your differential list?"

"Small bowel obstruction from adhesions," a young woman replied.

"You're absolutely right," I told her. "How do you manage this?"

"Operate,"

"No, not necessarily," I said. "Many of these cases can be treated successfully by passing a long tube through the nose down into the dilated bowel. Several days of suction may relieve the obstruction."

"What was her white blood count?"

"That's an excellent question. Her white count was elevated with a left shift. What does that mean? Anybody?"

"The bowel is being compromised by the obstruction," said the redhead.

"So what do you do in a case like this?"

"I think you have to operate right away to prevent gangrene of the bowel," he said.

"Yes, indeed. And this woman was scheduled for surgery the same day. So, how would you prepare her for surgery?"

"Give her IV fluids and insert a Levin tube to empty the stomach before administering anesthesia."

"Why bother emptying the stomach?"

"So that she won't vomit and aspirate gastric contents into her lungs."

"Good. You students have done your reading and that's important. But this woman did not have a tube passed into her stomach. She aspirated vomitus in the OR before the surgery began. The anesthesiologist responded and passed a tube into the stomach and sucked out 300 cc of fecaloid material. Then the surgeon operated on the woman. He found and cut an adhesion, which was causing the obstruction. But the woman's aspiration pneumonia was so severe that she died two days later."

"They should have operated a lot sooner," a young woman said.

"That's right," I said.

THE NEXT CASE DEALT with had several simple, but important, teaching points. "A 70-year-old man was admitted to a hospital for physiotherapy following reduction of a dislocated hip," I told the students. "He then developed abdominal distension, nausea and vomiting which was treated initially with Tigan. The distension continued and this additional X-ray was obtained."

I placed the picture on the view box and asked the students what they saw. When there was no answer, I pointed to a long tubular structure and asked, "What is this?"

"That must be his bowel filled with gas," a student replied.

"Of course," I said. "Large bowel or small?"

"I guess it's the large bowel. It starts in the right lower quadrant and goes up toward the liver and then turns to the left and then ends in the left upper quadrant."

"Large bowel it is," I said. "What's the name of the first part of the large bowel?"

"The cecum."

"That's right. Now, take this ruler and measure the diameter of the cecum."

"It's 13 centimeters."

"Is that normal?" I asked.

"Why, no, it's not. It's very dilated."

"It sure is. When the cecum gets to 10-to-12 centimeters, it's in danger of rupturing and the distension has to be relieved promptly. Mind you, this man's cecum is 13 centimeters. But can anybody tell me what's causing this distension?"

"How about a cancer of the colon?"

"Good answer! I'll put *Cancer of the Colon* at the top of our differential diagnosis list. What else might be causing this distension?"

"What was that syndrome you mentioned earlier?" a student asked. "The one where paralytic ileus affects just the large bowel?"

"It began with O-G," another student said. "Something like that."

"Ogilvie's Syndrome," I said. "That would be a good possibility in this man's age group. So let's make *Ogilvie's Syndrome* Number 2. But you can't tell the difference between a cancer and Ogilvie's Syndrome without X-raying the inside of the bowel with a barium enema or looking inside the bowel with a colonoscope. But do you think that a barium enema might be risky in this case?"

When there was no answer, I explained that there was a big risk. "Inserting barium into a colon that is already dilated to 13 centimeters might cause the bowel to rupture and spew barium and stool into the abdominal cavity. And that would cause a very severe infection called barium peritonitis."

"Then I guess a colonoscope would be safer," a student ventured.

"Yes, I'd say so, providing the doctor is careful not to pump a lot of air into the colon. The colonoscope would allow the doctor to see an obstructing cancer. And if there was no cancer, the instrument could be used to suck out all of the gas responsible for the dilated bowel."

I checked my notes on the case. "At this point," I told the students, "a surgical consult was requested. The surgical resident and his attending physician reviewed the same X-rays you are looking at right now. They decided to get a barium enema to look for a tumor.

"But take a look at this." I put another X-ray picture on the view box next to the first film. "At the time the barium enema was scheduled, the man's cecum had enlarged." I handed my ruler to another student and asked him to measure the enlarged cecum.

"My God!" he said. "It's 17 centimeters! And they went ahead and put barium up this poor guy's ass anyway?"

"They sure did," I said. "They gave him the barium enema and within just a few hours, the man's condition began to deteriorate rapidly. His abdomen became grossly distended. He went into shock and then cardiac arrest. He was resuscitated and rushed to the OR. What do you think they found?"

"A ruptured cecum," all the students answered.

"Absolutely correct. The right side of the man's colon had a huge tear in it. Large quantities of barium and stool were found throughout his abdomen. In spite of multiple surgeries, he died one month later from overwhelming sepsis."

"I'm amazed he lived that long," a student said.

"Me, too." I took a moment to erase the blackboard. "There's an important point to this man's story, one that you shouldn't take lightly. When you start practicing as doctors, don't ever give an enema – especially a barium enema – to a patient whose large bowel is greatly distended. You could kill your patient. This fellow's cause of death was listed as overwhelming sepsis. But we all know better, don't we? Don't ever forget what happened to him."

THAT AFTERNOON'S LAST CASE was that of a 43-year-old woman who underwent an abdominal hysterectomy because of abnormal uterine bleeding from fibroids.

"One day following surgery," I told the students, "the woman's abdomen became distended with gas. Can anyone tell me what has happened?"

A young woman asked: "Could this be a paralytic ileus, Dr. Kessler?"

"Yes, it could. You see, during abdominal surgery, the bowel is pushed aside to make room for the surgeon to see what he or she is trying to do. Manipulation of the bowel may cause temporary paralysis of the intestines, so that gas and fluid accumulate in the bowel and cause distension. How do you treat that?"

"IV fluids," she said. Another student added, "Don't feed the patient and pass a Levin tube."

"Good thinking. If you try to feed the patient, the distension gets worse. But this lady was given a liquid diet the first day. The next day she was put on a regular diet."

Several students groaned.

"Enemas, laxatives and suppositories did not help," I continued. "By Day Five, the woman's abdomen is huge and, when you tap it, it resonates like a drum. Even so, she's still being fed solid food and being considered for discharge."

A student interrupted. "What did her X-ray show?"

"X-rays had not yet been done."

"You're kidding!"

"No, unfortunately, I'm not. Now, by this time, the woman has a lot of abdominal pain. On Day Six, an IV is restarted and a Levin tube passed. By now, she's complaining of pain in the right upper quadrant and pain in the shoulder. What's happened?"

"The bowel has perforated, a young man said. " Did they finally get an X-ray?

"Yes, and it showed an enormous dilation of the colon and small bowel. It also showed lots of air surrounding the outside of the bowel. The woman's potassium was 3.0. Can anyone explain what that means?"

"Isn't that very low?" a student ventured.

"Right," I said. "Remember that not enough potassium can cause a paralytic ileus." The students bent over their notebooks. I waited until they had jotted down that information.

"Finally, a surgeon operated on the woman and discovered a small hole in her colon under her liver. Fortunately, there had not been any spillage of stool. The surgeon sutured the hole and drained the woman's abdomen. She recovered without incident. On Day 15, she was discharged from the hospital and went home. But, over the next two years, she had several bouts of small bowel obstruction. What caused that?"

All hands rose at once. "Adhesions!"

"Yes, adhesions," I said. "Eventually she had an episode that could not be relieved with a long tube. So an exploratory operation was performed. This revealed an adhesive band of scar tissue in the area of the previous perforation. That's what had been causing her multiple attacks of obstruction."

"And somebody got sued," said a student.

"Well," I said, "the woman and her husband asked a lawyer to investigate the possibility that her case had been mismanaged. Three local surgeons reviewed the case. They all agreed there had been negligence in the management of the woman's post-operative bloating. But all three were unwilling to testify."

"That's not hard to understand. They all worked in the same small community. The lawyer should have looked for an expert witness from somewhere else in the country. Instead, the lawyer diddled around and let the statute of limitations expire. And so the woman's doctors were off the hook."

I looked around the table. "I can see that you're disappointed," I said to them. "Yes, the doctors were off the hook. But not the small-town lawyer. He happened to be the brother of the gynecologist who had performed the woman's hysterectomy. The woman and her husband sued the lawyer for malpractice – and they won."

Several students shouted, "Hooray!"

19

KID STUFF

I'VE REVIEWED HUNDREDS of potential malpractice cases for attorneys, some of which involved children. Of all the cases sent to me for review, I found negligence in less than half. But in those cases where I found negligence which resulted in death, near-death, disfigurement or permanent physical damage, I detected a pattern of common mistakes.

In many cases, I found reluctance, procrastination and failure to call in a specialist for a consultation until it was too late. And far too many doctors tried to manage critical situations by telephone. That was true also of cases involving children. The children's cases, I found, had less to do with pediatrics than breaches of standards that apply to all medical specialties.

EXAMPLE: A TEN-YEAR-OLD GIRL was admitted to a hospital with typical symptoms of appendicitis. Unfortunately, her surgery was delayed for over 24 hours. It was bad enough that her appendix ruptured. The bigger problem was the inappropriate use of antibiotics before and after surgery.

The drugs chosen were not ones with track records that proved their efficacy against the variety of bacteria observed in a ruptured appendix. This mistake resulted in a prolonged illness and the need for several more operations to drain multiple intra-abdominal abscesses, to close a perforated stomach ulcer and to close a fecal fistula – a connection between the bowel and the skin. All those operations left the girl's abdomen crisscrossed with multiple ugly scars.

Several of the drugs she had been given were ototoxic. They're toxic to nerves that control hearing and are known to cause deafness, especially if they are used in combination. When using such drugs, it's necessary to monitor the blood level of the antibiotic and frequently test for hearing loss. That wasn't done in this girl's case.

Luckily, the child survived all these mistakes, but she ended up stone deaf with a seizure disorder. The pre-pubescent girl probably was rendered infertile because the severe infection in her belly most likely blocked her Fallopian tubes.

Her family filed a lawsuit which was settled for over $700,000 dollars. That sounded like a lot of money to my young students, but I don't think it was an excessive award. If the 10-year-old disfigured, deaf girl with slim chances of marriage lives to be 60, that award comes to $14,000 a year.

I doubt that any parents, knowing that their damaged child could out-live them, would ever advocate putting a cap on malpractice awards.

MOST OF MY PEDIATRIC experience came during the earlier years of my career: two months on the Pediatric Service during my internship, two years taking care of soldiers' children at the U.S. Army dispensary in France and four months of extensive training in Pediatric Surgery at Children's Hospital in Washington, D.C., when I was a surgical resident.

I also did a lot of pediatric surgery during my year in private practice in Ithica, New York. My patients at the VA Hospital in Manhattan were adults, of course, but I did participate in the care of infants and children at Bellevue Hospital.

Only gradually, as I reviewed case after case for lawyers, did I come to the realization that children's tragic stories followed the same pattern of mistakes I had been finding in the cases of adults: diagnosis and treatment by remote control, mismanagement of antibiotics, procrastination and failure to obtain early surgical consultations.

As my file of nightmare stories about dead and damaged children grew, I began sharing some of them with my students. It's never too early for young people hoping to become doctors to learn that infants and children are just as vulnerable to fatal stupidity as adults – probably more so.

I TOLD MY STUDENTS one story about a child who became a victim of remote-control medicine. The ten year-old boy's mother called a pediatrician when her child complained of abdominal pain. The doctor listened, asked a few questions, and then decided to treat the boy with antibiotics for one week. He did this over the phone without actually seeing the child.

My students usually found it hard to believe that the doctor never examined the boy. But he didn't, not until the week had passed. By that time, the boy's abdomen was as hard as a rock. His perforated appendix had spread pus all through his belly.

He was so sick that he damn near died. He would have if he hadn't been transferred to a university hospital. He was placed in the care of a nationally known pediatric surgeon who had to perform several operations to drain abscesses and resect part of the boy's stomach because of stress-ulcer bleeding. The little boy spent about six months in the hospital.

I traveled to the Midwest to testify for the boy and his family in that malpractice case. It ended with a hung jury – an outcome that never failed to shock my medical students.

"Why couldn't the jury agree on a verdict?" they'd ask and I'd reply, "The eminent pediatric surgeon who saved the boy's life testified in defense of the pediatrician who had put the boy in danger of death in the first place. The diagnosis of appendicitis, he stated in his testimony, can be difficult to make in the best of hands."

"Especially," snapped a young man, "if you make your diagnosis over the telephone!"

My students often made remarks like that, assuring me that they'd grasped the point of the story. A doctor should put down his phone, and go put his hands on the patient's belly and then make his diagnosis. It's really not all that difficult a diagnosis to make.

The boy's parents, as it turned out, were more demoralized by the testimony of the expert witness for the defense than the inability of the jury to reach a verdict. They decided to give up and accept an out-of-court settlement rather than go through a trial again.

ANOTHER CASE I PRESENTED to my students concerned a 14-year-old African-American boy who was admitted to a small hospital in Chicago complaining of a bellyache. He was seen by a surgeon in the late afternoon. The boy was tender in the right lower quadrant and had an elevated white blood count. The surgeon accurately diagnosed acute appendicitis and scheduled the surgery for ten o'clock the next morning.

The boy was placed on a ward and was given multiple shots of narcotics to relieve his pain and medicine to stop his vomiting. But he did not receive any intravenous fluids nor was a tube put in his stomach to stop the vomiting. He languished on this back ward all night. The nurses noted on his chart that he was breathing very rapidly. Early that morning, an orderly arrived to transport the boy to the operating room. He found the boy in his bed, dead.

An autopsy showed that the boy had undergone a splenectomy several months earlier because of a stab wound. Scar tissue from that surgery had caused a bowel obstruction. A short segment of his small bowel was gangrenous, or dead. The boy had died of severe acidosis from dead gut.

Students always asked if the boy could have been saved if he had been operated on sooner. My answer was always: "Yes, absolutely! Once a doctor diagnoses appendicitis, surgery should commence as quickly as possible, not at the convenience of the surgeon. The cause of the boy's death was procrastination."

And, I say to myself, perhaps stereotypic thinking. His parents' malpractice case was settled for peanuts. I wasn't surprised. The little boy was Black and his family was on welfare. I can't help suspecting that might have affected the judgment of the doctor and the nurses – not to mention the decision reached by the lawyers who negotiated the legal agreement on what the boy's life was worth: in this case, not much.

I HAVE NO WAY OF KNOWING how much (or how little) stereotypic thinking may have played a part in that case, but consider what happened to another child: the 11-year-old Rodriguez boy who went into surgery for the removal of his appendix which had ruptured.

The operation lasted one hour. He was taken to the recovery room with an IV running, an endotracheal tube in place and a nasogastric tube in his stomach. (Half of the recovery room staff was out to lunch at the time, by the way.)

One hour later and two hours after that, a large amount of vomitus tinged with blood was suctioned from the back of his throat. One of the RR nurses took care of it, but she didn't call a doctor. The nurse later noticed that the boy's breathing was shallow but, again, she didn't notify a doctor.

When I reviewed the case, I found that the boy's level of consciousness had never been entered in the recovery room record. Nor did the record show any post-op visits by the boy's anesthesiologist or surgeon. It did show that his endotracheal tube had been removed, but the record didn't indicate when or by whom.

Two and one half hours after entering the recovery room, the boy still had not awakened from the anesthesia. He went into cardiac arrest. A code was called. Ten minutes after the cardiac arrest, artificial ventilation through a new endotracheal tube was begun with an ambulatory bag.

That was nine minutes too late. The boy should have been ventilated immediately. About 15 to 20 minutes after the cardiac arrest, they gave the boy adrenalin and sodium bicarb (again, much too late). Twenty minutes after that, the boy's blood gases had a pH of 7.0, which was very low, and his PCO_2 was 54. That indicated that he was still retaining CO_2.

They didn't use electric shock because the boy's heartbeat returned after external cardiac massage. But the cardiac arrest and the ten-minute delay in ventilating the patient had guaranteed severe brain damage. You see, when this sort of thing occurs, the brain swells. Fluids need to be restricted. And you need to use drugs – such as steroids and Manitol – to reduce the swelling.

The boy wasn't given those drugs, but he was filled up with huge amounts of IV fluids for four hours – as much as 350 cc per hour. That would be enough to drown a child like the 11-year-old Rodriguez boy who weighed only about 90 pounds.

That first day in the hospital, he got a total of 5000 cc of IV fluid – twice as much as his body could handle. (That much fluid would increase brain swelling.) His chest X-ray was abnormal and that suggests aspiration, congestive failure or what's called "shock lungs".

The following day, two consultants suggested restricting the boy's fluids to 60 cc per hour and administering Manitol. But that consultation and advice came too late. The damage had been done. Three weeks later, the Rodriguez boy died.

It was a sad case with many mistakes. Here you had a boy who wasn't waking up from the anesthesia administered during surgery. It's most probable that this boy was hypoventilating because of the prolonged effect of the anesthetic agents. When that persists, the patient becomes anoxic – low in oxygen – and may vomit and aspirate and thus have a cardiac arrest. What this boy had needed was close observation by the nurses and the anesthesiologist.

If a patient is hypoventilating, the oxygen goes down and the CO_2 goes up. So this boy's endotracheal tube should not have been removed without first testing the blood gases. That would have shown whether or not they were ventilating the boy properly with adequate oxygen and that he was not retaining CO_2. The endotracheal tube should not have been removed. Actually, what the boy had needed was a respirator.

The family sued, of course. But their case was settled for $15,000. Why such a small amount?

The Rodriguez boy was one child in a large family that was on welfare and lived in the housing projects. Pragmatic lawyers considered that his chances of ever going to college were remote. They reasoned that it was not likely that he would have grown up to make a significant contribution to his family or to society.

In their eyes, his life was not worth as much as that of a white child from an affluent family. Bad enough that the boy died. Prejudice – whether conscious or unconscious – made the Rodriguez family's tragedy even worse.

Another factor in the bad outcome of the Rodriguez case that shouldn't be overlooked was the mismanagement of IV fluids. How much you give a patient recovering from surgery is calculated from the patient's age and weight. Miscalculating can be a fatal error that endangers all infants and children – rich or poor or in-between.

Family affluence, prestige or power cannot defend a child against stupid mistakes or avoidable errors.

WHEN MEDICAL STUDENTS ROTATE through pediatrics in the third or fourth year of their training, they learn that infants and small children have different IV requirements than adults. You don't have to be a rocket scientist to figure that out. You can tell just by looking. Infants and children are smaller than grown-ups. So, obviously, they need less IV fluids than adults.

In fact, they can't tolerate the same amount of fluid that adults can handle. If you give large quantities of IV fluids too rapidly to children – or very elderly patients, for that matter – you can overload them and cause heart failure or brain swelling. That is to say: you can kill them.

That was what I was telling my students on one typical day. "There's a pretty simple rule of thumb here," I said, nodding to one of the young women. "Can you put it into words?"

"Well, yes," she said. "Don't give little people as much IV fluid as you give big people. But it's not that simple, is it? Otherwise, you wouldn't be asking."

"You're right. In the real world there's always something I call an X-factor. X equals whatever it is that makes people act stupidly, something that causes health care professionals to lose sight of the obvious, such as the fact they're taking care of a child, not an adult.

"This is a story about a bright, happy seven-year-old little girl. She weighed 44 pounds. Except for frequent bouts of tonsillitis, her general health was good. Her family was white, affluent and professional, Her Dad was a doctor; her Mom was a nurse. They took their daughter to a general hospital to have her tonsils removed and they stayed with their little girl until she was taken to the OR for this routine operation. Her Mom and Dad had told her there was nothing to worry about and that she needn't be frightened. So she wasn't. Well, maybe a little bit.

"The little girl was put to sleep around 8:00 o'clock in the morning. The tonsillectomy began about 15 minutes later and lasted approximately 20 minutes. She arrived in the recovery room about 20 minutes later.

"Now, just before the girl was put to sleep, the anesthesiologist had hooked up an IV and a 500 cc bottle of IV fluid. The bottle was empty when the little girl got to the Recovery Room, so it was unhooked and replaced by a full 1,000 cc bottle. After 90 minutes, the little girl was awake enough to be moved to a regular hospital room – with the IV still attached.

"Start jotting down some figures," I told a young man. "The little girl was in the RR for an hour and a half during which time she received 200 cc of IV fluid from the 1,000 cc bottle. By 2:00 p.m., that bottle with the remaining 800 cc was finally empty. How much fluid had she received by then?"

The student looked up from the figures he'd been jotting down in his notebook. "She got 1,500 cc of IV fluid in about six and a half hours, Dr. Kessler. I get a rate of 230 cc per hour. That seems to be a lot for a little kid like her. What should it have been?"

"For a 44-pound child, the normal rate would be 60-70 cc per hour."

"She was getting way more than that! Didn't anybody notice anything wrong with her?"

"Well, yes and no. The little girl vomited several times during the day. That's not unusual after a tonsillectomy. Her nausea and vomiting was treated with Tigan suppositories on three occasions. Tigan, by the way, is a central nervous system depressant.

"Later in the afternoon, another IV bottle was connected to the girl's IV – a 500 cc bottle this time. Now, get this. According to the hospital record, over the next nine hours, the child received only 200 cc"

"That doesn't seem like a lot,"

"It isn't," I said, "But the little girl's mother said that her daughter got much more than 200 cc The mother's diary of events indicated that between 6:30 and 7:30 that evening, her daughter received 400 cc of fluid. She turned down the IV rate herself and told the floor nurse what had happened. She also wrote that her daughter had been voiding large amounts of urine all day long. What do you think caused that?"

"This is just a guess," said the young man, "but I think her kidneys were trying to get rid of the excess fluid."

"Right on," I told him. "Apparently – and this doesn't show up in the hospital record of fluids given – they gave her another 500 cc bottle of IV fluids after that, but how much the girl received from that bottle is unknown. At any rate, around 6:00 p.m., the child started to become lethargic.

"Two hours later, she vomited and wet the bed without waking up. A nurse called the doctor who had done the tonsillectomy – called him several times, in fact – and finally got to tell him about the girl's nausea and vomiting. He prescribed Tigan, over the phone, and advised the nurse to keep the child in the hospital overnight."

"Do they normally discharge tonsillectomy patients on the same day?"

"Nowadays, they do. Hospitals usually discharge most patients too soon. But that's not an issue here. What's more to the point is that this surgeon had not seen the little girl since he finished operating on her at 8:30 in the morning."

"Aren't doctors supposed to see their patients after they operate on them?"

"Absolutely! Surgeons should check their patient in the recovery room before leaving the OR area to be sure they're waking up properly, that no bleeding has occurred, and so on. And they're also supposed to check their patient again before they leave the hospital.

"By 11 o'clock that night," I continued, "the little girl's Mom was really upset. Her daughter was unconscious and she couldn't wake her up. Fifteen minutes later, the child had a grand mal seizure. The doctor finally arrived at midnight.

"By 1:30 a.m., the little girl was experiencing increased difficulty breathing. Her oxygen saturation was very low – around 50. Her blood gases showed a pH of 6.99 and her PO_2 was about 40. In short: the little girl was just about dead. She was intubated and placed on a respirator. That caused a slight improvement in her blood gases, but a chest X-ray showed a lot of fluid in her lungs. It wasn't until this point that the doctor called for a pediatric consult!

"The pediatric specialist quickly determined that the child had been overloaded with IV fluids. That, he said, had caused the pulmonary edema —the fluid in the lungs – and had also caused the little girl's brain to swell. Her body temperature had dropped to 94 degrees.

"The little girl was transferred from the general hospital to a children's hospital. Shortly after she arrived there, her Mom and Dad got the bad news: their little girl's pupils were dilated and they were not reacting to light. Because of excessive swelling, her brain stem had herniated through her foramen magnum.

Her parents were medical professionals and knew only too well what this doctor was telling them. The swelling had pushed their daughter's brain stem out through the base of her skull. She was brain dead."

A young woman broke the silence. "My God! The poor little kid went to have her tonsils out and those incompetent bastards killed her! I hope something really bad happened to them!"

"I don't know about the individuals involved. I do know that the hospital took a big hit, but not in the way you might imagine. That's because this little girl's parents were truly remarkable. Most people would have been consumed with grief and anger and the urge for revenge, but these parents decided to be positive and charitable.

"They assembled their family members to see the little girl for one last time and say their good-byes. Then they gave their permission to shut down all the devices that were keeping the child's body functioning even though her brain was dead.

"Her Mom and Dad sat by her empty bed long after orderlies had taken her body to an operating room where surgeons took her vital organs so that a few seriously ill children could have a chance to keep on living.

"Her father wrote in his diary: 'This may in some inadequate way make up for her senseless death.' He wrote that entry at 7:30 in the morning, just two days after the little girl had walked into the hospital for a routine tonsillectomy.

"The parents, of course, took legal action against the hospital and the surgeon. I never did learn if their lawsuit was successful or if it ever did get to court. Their lawyer, I know, was eventually sued for allowing the statute of limitations to run out on four cases he was handling. I can only hope the parents' case was not one of them.

"Be that as it may, their little girl's story spread like wildfire through the community, and the damage to the hospital was immediate. Doctors in the area, especially pediatricians, simply stopped sending their patients to that hospital.

"Now, a hospital can gradually replace the money it has lost in a malpractice case, but it can never completely recover its good name. No matter what changes it makes, it's always going to be known in its community as the hospital where something terrible happened to a seven-year-old girl."

After a few moments, a young woman spoke up. "I don't understand how simple operations can go so wrong," she said.

"This simple operation went wrong because people who should know better made stupid decisions and disastrous mistakes," I replied.

"I know you're all gung-ho right now and you can't imagine that you'll ever become that kind of a doctor. Well, just wait until you have to start paying off your student loans – on an intern's salary. Wait until personal and financial problems start closing in on you. Then you'll understand. It happens in every profession, in any business, on any job, in any relationship. What we're all up against is human nature.

"Somewhere along the line, people get distracted and lose their sense of commitment to what they're engaged in doing. They begin to forget they're dealing with other people who depend on them.

"They become bored, indifferent, impatient, and less and less attentive to details. They begin to look for short cuts and take unnecessary risks. Eventually they make mistakes that cause really bad things to happen to other people – job loses, divorces, foreclosures, traffic accidents, oil spills, plane crashes.

"As for medical people like us? We're not immune. Make a couple of mistakes in a hospital or a private medical practice and somebody winds up dead or permanently disabled. It doesn't take much for us to ruin a person's whole life."

I LOOKED AT MY WATCH. I had given my students a break. Now they were returning and taking their seats at the table. "Get ready for another case of bad medicine," I told them and waited until they had all settled down.

"Now," I said, "we're going to turn our attention to a 14-year-old girl who developed right-sided abdominal pain while she was away from home during the summer months. While she was out-of-town, she was diagnosed as a case of VD and treated with a course of penicillin,"

I paused, waiting for a question or two, but the students remained silent. I told them that they would need to review the previous week's discussion of VD and waited while they skimmed through their notebooks. A young man found a page that gave him a clue about the right question to ask.

"What sort of VD did she have?"

"PID – pelvic inflammatory disease."

"Gonorrhea in a 14-year-old?

"Sure," I said. "It's entirely possible. I've seen 14-year-olds who were sexually active. In fact, I've delivered babies from 14-year-old girls."

"Really? Where was that?"

"In Washington," I said. "I did my internship at D.C. General Hospital. They delivered 500 babies a month at that hospital when I was there."

"But you're a general surgeon," young woman said. "How many babies have you delivered?"

"Over 300," I said. "I delivered eight babies in one eight hour shift at D.C. General. And there was one night when I delivered a 14-year-old's first child and her 28-year-old mother's eighth. It's been a long time since my last delivery. That was a baby boy when I was in the Army in France. But you've got me off the track. Are there any questions about the case at hand?"

"What color was her vaginal discharge?"

"At this point, she didn't have a discharge."

"How's that possible?" asked Ira.

"Well, it's a remote possibility," I said. "But I've never seen a case of gonorrhea that didn't produce a yellow vaginal discharge. The cultures of this girl's vaginal secretions failed to grow out gonococcus or any other bug, such as Chlamydia, that causes VD. But they treated her with penicillin anyway. And after two weeks went by, she returned to her home in New Jersey.

"She was still very ill. The following day, she was admitted to a hospital with a temperature of 104 and a white blood count of 17.6. Her abdominal pain had increased and was now associated with a vaginal discharge."

"What was the color and odor of her vaginal discharge?"

"It was muddy in color and it produced a foul odor that smelled of feces."

"Had she had an illegal abortion?" asked one of the young women. "I mean, not in a real medical facility?"

"That's an excellent question," I said. "We know back-room dirty abortions can result in a PID with a mixed bag of bugs that cause a foul vaginal discharge. But the answer is no. She hadn't had an abortion, legal or illegal. At any rate, her home-town doctors gave her 10-million units of penicillin because they thought her problem was secondary to gonorrhea."

"Then how did they explain the foul smell," she asked.

"Her physicians didn't appreciate the significance of the odor. Nor the significance of a large mass they palpated in her pelvis. It extended up into her abdomen and ended above her belly button. The doctors concluded that it was a tube-ovarian abscess secondary to VD, involving the tubes and ovary."

"Did they culture the vaginal discharge?"

"Yes," I answered, "and it grew out multiple bacteria found in the bowels."

"Did gonococcus grow out, too?

"No, never," I answered. "But the culture results did not come back from the lab until after surgery was performed. I should add that before they operated they also considered a ruptured appendix as a possible cause for this patient's problems."

"That should have been Number One on their list!"

"You're right, but it wasn't," I said. "Two days in the hospital and 10-million units of penicillin didn't improve her condition. She wasn't getting any better, so she was finally taken to the OR for an exploratory laparotomy.

"The surgeon discovered a huge abscess that adhered to all the adjacent organs – including the bowel, the fallopian tubes, the ovaries and the uterus. The abscess was opened and drained. It yielded almost two quarts of foul-smelling, dirty, brown pus. Now, what does that foul odor suggest to all of you?"

"It's caused by multiple coliform bacteria."

"Such as?"

"Bacteroides!" Several students had the correct answer." Very good," I said. "Now, while evacuating the abscess, the surgeons found a fecalith. What's a fecalith, again?"

"A small piece of shit," mumbled Ira.

"We prefer to use the term 'stool,' Ira. So, what does the presence of a fecalith in an abscess suggest to you?"

"That there is a hole someplace in the bowel," he replied.

"That's correct. Stool is only found inside the bowel. It doesn't come from the tubes or leak out of the uterus or the gall bladder. Only from the bowel! Has everybody got that?" All the students nodded, so I continued. "The surgeons also found a hole in the colon where the appendix would normally be attached. What does that suggest to you?"

"She has a perforated appendix?"

."Most likely," I said. "What's the most common cause of appendicitis?"

"A fecalith getting stuck in the base of the appendix."

"Right on! So what should the surgeons do now?"

"Remove the appendix."

"No, drain the abscess. The surgeons couldn't find the appendix, remember? So what should they do about that hole in the colon? The hole where the appendix should have been?"

"Sew up the hole," one student said.

"No," I said. "The sutures probably wouldn't hold in all that infection. They should put a tube in the hole and bring the colon to the outside as in a controlled fecal fistula. In this case, it would be called a cecostomy, since the tube would be in the part of the colon called the cecum. And then, they should call it a day."

"Could you culture the pus?" the young woman in scrubs asked.

"Absolutely," I replied. "I'm glad you brought that up. They did that. What do you think the cultures showed?"

"Multiple colonic bacteria, of course."

"Of course," I said, "and no gonococcus was found. Now, tell me this: how does an infection from a ruptured appendix or bowel get into the vagina?"

"It travels through the Fallopian tubes and the uterus. It finally reaches the vagina where it exits out as drainage."

"You know, it's too damn bad you students weren't in charge of this girl's case. Because, you see, her surgeons proceeded to perform a total abdominal hysterectomy which was difficult and bloody, to say the least. The girl was in shock throughout most of the procedure. She required five blood transfusions and over 3,000 cc of IV fluids. What's your opinion on this?"

The students just stared at me. A soft-spoken young woman finally responded. "But, why?" she said. "Why the hysterectomy?"

"Beats me," I said. "It appears that these surgeons believed they were dealing with a tubo-ovarian abscess, secondary to VD. That was sheer folly, of course, considering the evidence before them. At any rate, the dissection they had to perform spread the infection throughout the girl's abdomen.

"During the next two months, she underwent drainage of another large abscess and endured the creation of a colostomy because of a perforation in the large bowel. She was critically ill much of the time and she received an additional 15 blood transfusions because of stress ulcer bleeding.

"Her antibiotic management was haphazard and it often consisted of a combination of drugs such as Gentamycin, Kantrex and Neomycin. Do you have any problem with those antibiotics?" I asked the students.

"They can cause deafness, can't they?" one replied.

"Yes, especially if used in combination. How do you try to avoid a hearing loss from the use of antibiotics? Anyone?"

"You measure the blood levels of the drugs and you give frequent audiometer tests to check the patient's hearing."

"Correct," I said. "In this girl's case, an audiometer test was done only once."

"So, she's deaf now?"

"Yes, she's deaf," I said. "And she gets hot flashes from the loss of her ovaries. And she's sterile. A severe case of appendicitis, you see, can result in sterility caused by the infection blocking the tubes. In her case, the pathology report revealed that both tubes were patent and that the infection was on the outside of the tubes and uterus.

"Nevertheless, an expert witness reviewed the case on behalf of the two doctors responsible for the surgery and concluded that '*they were free from any deviation from accepted standards ... were diligent ... and performed life-saving surgery and antibiotic management.*' What do you think of that assessment?"

"The expert witness was an asshole or a liar, or both," said Ira. "What did he have to say about the foul-smelling discharge and fecalith?"

"He never mentioned those issues." I said.

"Law school, here I come," said Ira. It was one of the remarks he often made. But this time, nobody laughed.

"I want you all to think about this girl's case." I said, "and remember it if you ever find yourself in a similar situation. If something looks like stool, smells like stool and feels like stool, you should conclude that it is stool and can only come from the bowels."

MOST STUDENTS LEFT the conference room, but Ira and a tall young woman named Susan stayed to talk with me. I'd noticed that Susan tended to take cases personally. She'd been an exemplary anatomy student in her first year of medical school. Now, in her third year, she had let her emotions surface during some other cases we had been reviewing. Nothing wrong with that, I thought. She was going to become a fine, compassionate doctor someday.

"The girl's family," said Ira. "They sued the bastards, didn't they, Dr. Kessler?"

"Yeah, the family sued. The two surgeons got off real easy. They settled out of court for $350,000 apiece. But the doctor who treated her for two weeks using penicillin without any evidence of gonorrhea? He lost at trial and the jury awarded the girl one million dollars. Do you think that was excessive, Susan?"

Susan shook her head slowly. "The poor kid became deaf and post-menopausal at the age of 14," she said quietly. "She'll probably never get married. She'll probably outlive her parents and end up all alone with no one to care for her. No, I don't think a million dollars was excessive at all."

20

A FEDERAL CASE

IT'S NOT A GOOD DAY when the least worrisome item on my schedule is a visit by a U.S. Attorney. He'd made an appointment to discuss a case that had been dropped in his lap for investigation and now here he was sitting in my office.

The case involved a patient in a our V.A. hospital, a veteran who had undergone a lymph node biopsy in his neck. A chief resident had supervised a junior resident during the procedure which was performed under local anesthesia. An enlarged lymph node was removed for diagnostic testing for cancer. But something had gone wrong and now the veteran was suing the government.

"It appears that your doctors accidentally cut a nerve that controls shoulder movements," said the U.S. attorney, getting right to the point.

"That's right," I answered. "The doctors damaged the spinal accessory nerve. That's the nerve that controls the trapezius muscle on the side of the neck."

The attorney checked off something on his yellow legal notepad. "What happens when the muscle is not working properly?"

"Significant neurological defect," I answered. "That's exactly what you are observing in this patient. The shoulder sags. There's shoulder pain. The person has trouble raising the shoulder. The trapezius muscle atrophies because it is now paralyzed. Because of this muscle atrophy, the neck looks lop-sided. Furthermore, the shoulder blade protrudes out from the back. That's a defect we call a winged scapula."

"Can this be fixed?"

I shook my head. "It's very unlikely in this patient's case because the trapezius muscle has already atrophied. Even if a spinal accessory nerve is repaired soon after an injury, the results are poor. And, in this case, the trapezius muscle has been atrophied for six months."

"How could the nerve get damaged in such a minor procedure? It *is* a minor procedure, isn't it, Doctor?"

"Not really. A lymph node biopsy in the neck should never be considered a minor procedure because the spinal accessory nerve is located just beneath the lumps that are being removed. Unfortunately, the mistake made in this case was a mistake many surgeons make."

"Does the nerve get cut?"

"It's either cut or crushed with a clamp or burned by a cautery used to control bleeding."

"So exactly what happened in this case?"

"I don't know for sure," I said. "But I can tell you that they used a cautery which should *never* be used near an important nerve. Mistakes like this one usually occur because the surgeon has forgotten his anatomy and is operating in a plane that is too deep."

"So tell me, Doctor, how can we defend this case?"

"We can't. It's indefensible."

"I'm not sure my bosses will want to hear that."

"Then give it to them straight and simple. A mistake was made and there's no way to wiggle out of that. So settling out of court is the right thing to do. It won't involve a substantial money loss, by the way. The poor guy has AIDS and I'm afraid he doesn't have very long to live. So if your superiors don't buy the idea that settling is the right thing to do, you can make the argument that it's cost effective."

The attorney gave me a stricken look.

"I'm sure they'll follow your recommendation, but they'll have a few more questions. For example: when did the doctors become aware of the problem?"

"Not until the patient showed up in our clinic complaining about his shoulder."

"Shouldn't the problem have been recognized in the OR?"

"Probably, but technical mistakes often go unrecognized by surgeons. I'd say 75% of the time."

"Where are you getting that figure from, Doctor?"

"From years of experience reviewing potential malpractice cases for law firms."

"How many years?

"About 20."

"Have you reviewed cases like this before?"

"About a dozen, at least."

"In those cases, did the surgeons recognize the injuries in the OR?"

"Not once," I said. "And that's despite the fact that most of the patients remembered that their shoulder had twitched violently during the procedure."

"You found that significant?"

"Well, let me explain. As the relatively small spinal accessory nerve is being traumatized, it sends electrical signals to the trapezius muscle. That causes the muscle to contract. The patients were aware of that sudden reaction in the cases I reviewed but, for some reason, the surgeons were not."

"Did any of those patients undergo nerve repair?"

"Only one. But the repair was attempted five months too late and it wasn't successful."

"So you'd say it's a really serious injury?"

"For the patients, it's devastating. They wind up with chronic pain and a gross physical deformity, to boot."

"Did any of those cases you reviewed ever go to trial?"

"No, they all settled. Wisely, in my opinion."

"One last question, Doctor. How could this sort of injury be avoided?"

"Well, I seriously doubt that any patients are going to say, 'Doctor, please spare my spinal accessory nerve when you remove this lump from my neck.' But, if I had *my* way, every surgeon would be put on notice to review the anatomy before going into the operating room."

The U.S. attorney stowed his legal pad in his briefcase, thanked me for my time, shook my hand and left my office. That was the last I heard from the Federal government about the case. As it turned out, the patient died of AIDS a few months later.

The resident who had messed up his shoulder made no more serious mistakes while she was at our hospital. She completed the rest of her residency with flying colors and she went on to become an outstanding surgeon with a particular interest in anatomy.

I don't know what kind of an impression I made on the U.S. attorney that day. He seemed to have had no doubts about my medical skill and expertise, but then he had no access to my appointment calendar and had no way of measuring my anxiety level. It was through the roof because the next item on my agenda read: "M&M, Bellevue, 4:00 pm."

THE LAW REQUIRES HOSPITALS to review every case in which there has been a death or complication of treatment and New York University holds its weekly Morbidity and Mortality conferences on the surgical service at Bellevue Hospital on Manhattan's East Side.

For the physician who has made a serious error, the M&M conference can be a humiliating and sometimes brutal experience. The doctor has to present the case in question to a large group of surgeons, residents, medical students and nurses. The doctor must stand alone as members of the faculty criticize, but seldom praise, the way the case was handled. That afternoon one of the cases on the M&M agenda was mine.

As I walked along First Avenue toward Bellevue, I recalled some earlier conferences where physicians had their egos deflated by their peers.

"The patient's heart may have stopped on Saturday," one critic told the assemblage, "but he died on Tuesday when the wrong operation was done, again on Wednesday when he was allowed to become dehydrated and he died a third time when the wrong antibiotic was used. For God's sake, it would have been easier to just pick up a .45 and shoot him!"

The younger doctors call this weekly exercise "the Murder & Mayhem conference." And with good reason: no one is immune to blistering critiques at an M&M. I recalled one verbal shot fired at a female doctor – a Catholic missionary nun who was a chief resident at Bellevue. She was scheduled to rejoin her missionary order in Africa, but before her departure she was summoned to defend one of her cases.

A crusty old surgeon, noted for his skill and acid tongue, told the nun: "If you make this sort of mistake when you get back to Africa, Sister, your patients are likely to boil you in a big black pot and have you for dinner." With any luck, the old fart might be home sick and not available to critique *my* performance during this day's M&M.

I tried to squelch my feelings of impending doom and rode the hospital elevator up to the large conference room on the 15th floor. It's a room that can hold well over 100 people. It was not filled to capacity, thank goodness. I took a seat and started pulling myself together.

The true purpose of the M & M conference, I told myself, is salutary: to help other doctors avoid making the same mistake you have made. And to make sure the offending physician doesn't make the same mistake twice. That was fine with me, of course. I was perfectly willing to admit my mistake, but I thought hard about how I could dodge the slings and poisoned arrows of professional ego-deflators. I decided to assume the role of teacher and defuse my more hostile colleagues with some preemptive self-criticism.

The Chairman of the Department of Surgery entered the room and the M&M conference began. "Let's start with case Number Four from the VA Hospital," the chairman announced. "The bile duct injury." The young resident I had supervised on this case stood up and marched to the podium. If he was nervous, he did not show it.

"This," he said clearly and precisely, "is a case of a 55-year-old male who came to the VA hospital ER vomiting blood and passing blood per rectum. He gave a 35-year history of heavy drinking. He was emaciated, jaundiced and his liver was enlarged. He was in shock with a blood pressure of 60/0 when first seen.

"After he was resuscitated with IVs and three blood transfusions, he was endoscoped which revealed bleeding varices in the lower esophagus. A Blakemore tube was passed into the esophagus and the bleeding was controlled by balloon tampanade. When the balloons were deflated six hours later, the bleeding promptly recurred. IV vasopressin failed to stop the bleeding and the balloons were re-inflated.

"When the bleeding occurred again, a decision was made to do an emergency porta-caval shunt. Upon entering the abdomen, it was noted that the gall bladder was infected and contained hundreds of small gallstones. There were dilated veins around the gall bladder secondary to portal hypertension.

"It was decided to perform the shunt first in order to lower the pressure in the veins before taking on the infected gall bladder. An umbilical vein catheterization was done and revealed a portal pressure of 45 cm. – the normal being 10-15 cm.

"After an end-to-side porta-caval shunt was performed, the portal pressure dropped to 20 cm. and the dilated veins around the gall bladder were greatly reduced. We then planned to do a cholecystectomy with the intent of also exploring the common bile duct because of the jaundice and multiple small stones. During the dissection, a 3-mm. duct, which was presumed to be the cystic duct, was clamped, cut and ligated.

"After further dissection, it became clear that the duct we had cut was the main bile duct. This was repaired over a T-tube. There were no stones in the bile duct. Post-operatively, the patient did well for the first three-to-four days. But he then became lethargic, confused and disoriented. This progressed to full blown hepatic and renal failure and he died in coma 12 days following surgery."

The chairman dismissed the resident who left the podium and returned to his seat. "Dr. Kessler," said the chairman, "would you care to comment?"

"Yes, thank you." I took my place at the podium. "The key word in my colleague's presentation is '*presumed.*' We presumed that a small duct was the cystic duct. A surgeon should *never* presume. In my years of practice, I have never seen a bile duct that small. But, so what?

"I teach anatomy and each year I give a lecture on the liver and gall bladder. Each year I explain to the students all the variations in the blood vessels and bile ducts around the gall bladder. There are so many variations that I tell the students that there's no such thing as *normal* anatomy around the gall bladder. And I tell them that a surgeon should never cut a damn thing until he or she is absolutely sure of the identity of the structure to be clamped and cut.

"Now this is a basic rule that all surgeons should follow. But my colleague and I broke that rule and there's no excuse for it. Once I realized that we had cut the common bile duct, I experienced a sick feeling in the pit of my stomach. I knew that I had screwed up – big time!"

The room was quiet. No sarcastic remarks. At least, not yet.

"As we all know," I went on, "an injured bile duct can be a disaster for the patient months or even years later. Scar tissue forms and causes obstructions to the flow of bile. This can lead to infections in the liver and eventually – in some cases – cirrhosis. About 50% of bile duct injuries require additional surgeries and even then the patients may, in time, die from cirrhosis. This patient, however, didn't live long enough to develop any problems with his bile ducts.

"Our error with the bile duct was serious and inexcusable, but it was not the cause of death. The patient already had severe cirrhosis and he died of liver failure. An emergency shunt in a patient like that is associated with a high mortality rate. That's it," I said. There was more I could have added, but I thought it prudent to stop right there.

"Was this patient a Childs Class C patient?" asked the chairman.

"Yes, he was. A long-time heavy drinker with cirrhosis, a high-risk patient. A Childs Class C, to be sure. Most of our alcoholic patients at the VA are very poor risks, but we won't do a shunt if the patient has evidence of liver failure before surgery, such as confusion and disorientation – what we call encephelopathy. This patient's liver had not yet failed."

"What is the expected mortality from emergency shunts in poor risk patients?"

"Nationwide it's about 55%"

"What has been your experience?"

"About one third of our shunts have been done as an emergency procedure and we have lost 45%."

"How many shunts have you yourself done?"

"At least 120 porta-caval shunts and 15 to 20 meso-caval shunts."

"Well, I think you've covered it all," said the chairman. "Does anybody else have a question for Dr. Kessler?"

I held my breath and waited, but none of the sharks in the conference room took the bait. "Very well," said the chairman. He consulted his agenda. "Let's hear about the gunshot wound to the heart."

I had intended to leave as quickly as possible, but that gunshot stopped me in my tracks. When I was a resident at Washington Hospital Center in D.C., our ER had received five people who had been *stabbed* in the heart. We had saved four of those stabbing victims, but lost the fifth.

But I'd never treated a gunshot wound to the heart. So I returned to my seat and gave my full attention to the young resident at the podium. He had been on duty one night in the Bellevue emergency room when an ambulance crew brought in a man who had been shot in the heart. The man actually survived.

The young doctor's detailed presentation confirmed my oft-stated opinion that a good trauma team can accomplish great deeds. I've often said that if I was ever attacked or seriously injured, I hoped it would happen on East 25th Street near First Avenue because being delivered to the residents at the Bellevue Hospital ER would be my best chance for staying alive.

As a matter of fact, that's exactly where I was taken when I had a heart attack while putting this book together. Two doctors who took care of me were former Bellevue residents and students of mine. The reader can safely assume that I survived.

I MANAGED TO AVOID shark attacks at that M&M conference, but I've never been able to put the bile duct mistake out of my mind for very long. That's probably just as well.

Over the years that followed, I reviewed a dozen cases of bile duct injury for law firms. In half of those cases, the surgeon did not recognize the injury at the time. Six injuries occurred during laparoscopic surgery and six during open cholecystectomy. The common duct was repaired in seven cases. Five cases required the suturing of the small bowel to the liver (hepato-jejunostomy). Four cases required multiple operations and two patients eventually developed cirrhosis of the liver and died of hemorrhage from esophageal varices.

Of the 12 cases, only one went to trial. The surgeon was successfully defended by very competent lawyers. That's often the way things work out.

21

DID SOMEBODY SAY "CHEERS"?

SEVERAL YEARS AGO, one of the medical schools in the New York City area asked me to speak at a three-day seminar on alcoholism and drug addiction. That seminar, I found out, would be the only instruction on alcohol and drug abuse those medical students would receive during their entire four-year course of studies. That didn't surprise me. Even today, it's about par for the course nationally.

In my opinion, it's a serious deficiency in any medical school's curriculum. If you consider the immense amount of death and damage that's directly and indirectly caused by substance abuse. It's probably this country's biggest health problem and the one most misunderstood by most Americans – including those in the medical profession.

Not many doctors want to be bothered with drunks and drug addicts. For one thing, they can't be counted on to pay their bills. But I think the real reason doctors tend to avoid dealing with them is that they don't have the training to treat them properly. Some doctors never even learned how to make an accurate diagnosis.

That's understandable. When I was in medical school, I was taught about cirrhosis of the liver and other diseases caused by alcohol. But I received no training whatsoever about the *disease* of alcoholism. Back then, we weren't even taught that it was a disease.

It's no wonder that most doctors of my generation didn't know much, if anything, about how to diagnose or treat alcoholism. I certainly didn't, not until I left private practice in Ithaca to become a full-time surgeon and researcher at the VA Hospital in New York City. That's where I got my first real education in alcohol and drug addiction. There and at nearby Bellevue Hospital.

I joined the VA hospital staff in 1964 and my first job was supervising the residents who were taking care of patients in a 40-bed ward. When our hospital became officially affiliated with New York University Hospital in 1967, NYU's residents and third-year medical students began rotating through my surgical service for 12-week periods.

Time passed quickly and I settled comfortably in my new career. I was doing lots of teaching and lots of research, publishing three research papers per year and presenting my papers at national medical meetings. In short, I had found what I had been looking for – and a good deal more.

At a VA hospital or a big-city medical facility like Bellevue, a doctor constantly confronts the physical and psychological damage that war and economic hardship inflict on human beings. There are plenty of last-stage alcoholics and drug addicts for a doctor to treat and a medical researcher to observe. So, almost by accident, I became somewhat of an expert on drugs and alcohol – with enough scientific papers to prove it.

Bellevue Hospital was part of the NYU system, so I served there as well as an attending physician. I supervised the Bellevue residents during emergency surgeries, at least a couple of times a month. So I was keeping busy.

If memory serves, there was hardly a single Christmas or New Years Eve when my presence wasn't required in the VA Hospital's OR. Not that I complained; I liked being called up in an emergency. I enjoyed taking a first-year resident through an operation step by step. I got great satisfaction when a senior resident began requiring less and less assistance. I was proud when one of my chief residents could manage an average case, and delighted when the young doctor could operate confidently and independently a good deal of the time. Over the years at Bellevue and the VA, I performed operations or assisted residents doing surgery literally thousands of times.

The most difficult cases were alcoholics who were bleeding. Their surgery consisted of shunting the blood around the liver.

This porta-caval shunt was often technically difficult and bloody. Whenever this operation was needed, I was the one who was called. For 10 years, I averaged about one per month.

Sometimes I'd be able to talk a chief resident through this procedure, but most times I'd have to do much of the operation myself. Very few surgeons have done a porta-caval shunt; but because of where I worked, I had the opportunity to perform about 150.

For years, I watched residents and attending physicians treating the physical damage caused by the excessive use of alcohol and other drugs. I became aware that, more often than not, they failed to refer their patients to an appropriate program for ongoing treatment of their problem, such as Alcoholics Anonymous, Narcotics Anonymous or a rehabilitation program. So, in 1990, I began reviewing the medical records of patients admitted to the VA hospital's surgical service.

I WANTED TO DETERMINE what percentage of our patients had an addiction problem, whether it was responsible for the illness leading to admission and whether they were referred to an on-going treatment program for their substance abuse. In 1994, after reviewing 600 consecutive admissions, I was able to report the results at the annual meeting of the Research Society on Alcoholism that was held that year on the Hawaiian island of Maui.

Two hundred ten (35%) of those 600 surgical admissions gave a history of alcoholism or addiction to other drugs. Thirty-one (15%) were drug and alcohol free. Eighty-eight (42%) were being hospitalized because of a drug or alcohol related illness. Thirty-one (15%) had received detoxification treatment in the past, but only one had received treatment in a rehabilitation facility.

I found that the hospital's primary focus was on treating the disease or the problem that was responsible for the admission. Patients admitted for elective surgery who were still drinking were first detoxed in the hospital for several days to avoid serious post-operative alcohol withdrawal syndromes, such as delirium tremens.

At the time of discharge, a few of the patients were advised to go to AA. But long-term management was seldom addressed. Most patients never received long-term follow-up to deal with their addictions. I concluded that surgeons had to become more involved with their alcoholic patients and see to it that they were referred to the appropriate facility, clinic or recovery program.

I ENJOYED MY TIME on the beautiful island of Maui where I presented my research: (Kessler, R.E., Substance Abuse in a General Surgical Population: The Surgeon's Responsibility. Alcoholism: Clin. and Exp. Research 18:497: April – 1994.) Sitting through the entire conference was another matter.

I didn't learn much about alcoholism. Quite the contrary. I had to listen politely to an enormous amount of bullshit. Who would have possibly guessed that rats maintained on a diet of alcohol did not learn as quickly as rats fed a normal diet? Or that those freshmen college students who drank too much scored poorly on their exams?

Or that injury on ski slopes was more likely to occur if a skier had been imbibing alcohol? (I had to give that guy credit for convincing somebody to give him a grant to spend time at a ski resort doing research on the obvious.)

The results of some other research project purported to show that "the severity of injuries treated in emergency rooms was directly proportional to the amount of alcohol consumed." I appreciated having my own ER impressions confirmed by hard data, but the researcher lost me when he concluded with a suggestion that people needed to be taught how to control their drinking and to drink safely.

That would be sensible advice for skiers who are not alcoholics; but our nation's graveyards are filled with alcoholics (skiers and non-skiers alike) who have tried to drink safely.

What are the odds that an alcoholic can learn to drink safely? I'd say that about one alcoholic in 3,000 might succeed in achieving "moderate" or "social" drinking status. The problem is that, like other progressive diseases, alcoholism doesn't get better; it gets worse. So I made it a point that the medical students who rotated through my surgical service at the VA hospital got a good look at how bad "worse" can be.

SEVERAL TIMES A WEEK, I made rounds with the VA hospital's residents, nurses and students. And, once every week, I'd gather my medical students on the surgery ward for their own show-and-tell exercise. We'd walk from room to room and each student would present at least one case for discussion.

The group on this particular morning was made up of students who were completing their second week of surgical rotation. They were eager to learn and listened intently as one young woman presented the patient she had been caring for: a middle-aged veteran who had become a heroin addict during his tour of duty in Vietnam.

He'd been skin-popping and shooting up intravenously and had developed cellulitis – a serious infection in one of his legs which was red, slightly tender to touch and twice the size of his normal leg. His IV, she told her fellow students, contained a broad-spectrum antibiotic and was running into the patient through a subclavian-vein catheter.

"Does he have a fever?" I asked her.

"No, he doesn't."

"Is his white blood count elevated?"

"It was when he came in two days ago, but it's almost normal now."

"And has his leg gotten any better?"

"Oh, yes! It looked really awful two days ago!"

"And what's being done to treat his addiction?"

"He's on methadone," she said. "The plan is to wean him off it over several weeks."

"And what's the plan once the infected leg heals?"

"He'll be transferred up to the rehab ward for long-term rehabilitation."

"I'm absolutely amazed!" I said. "We're actually treating addiction properly these days. And it's only taken us a few thousand years to get to this point."

"Why couldn't this patient have been treated on an outpatient basis?" a young man asked. "Couldn't the ER have sent him home with antibiotics?"

"That's the way cellulitis is treated by most doctors," I told him. "That's because the HMOs and insurance companies usually won't approve admission to the hospital for cellulitis unless the patient is desperately ill. There are problems with that approach.

"Most of these cases are seen in alcoholics and drug addicts who have depressed immune systems and are infected with multiple or resistant bacteria. Most of the antibiotics needed to treat these infections can only be given intravenously – and that requires hospitalization.

"Also, if you send active alcoholics or drug addicts home with instructions to return at a later date, they probably won't return. They'll continue to drink or drug. They can't help it; that's the way they are. You won't see them until they're desperately ill again. So it's best to admit them to the hospital when they first show up. That way their infection and addiction can be treated at the same time."

I told the students about a heroin addict who checked into an ER with a severe case of cellulitis in the leg. He was sent home with a prescription for one of the penicillins and told to return in one week. He showed up three days later with gas gangrene of the leg caused by anaerobic bacteria which is only susceptible to certain intravenous antibiotics. His leg was amputated above the knee.

"I suppose he sued the doctor," a young man said.

"He did, but he accepted a settlement – a small one – rather than go through a trial where he'd be trashed for being a drug addict."

As I led the group along the hallway, I noticed that one of my students, a young man named Angus, was unusually quiet this morning. He didn't look well. His eyes were puffy and bloodshot.

He seemed to be hiding behind the other students, trying not to be noticed. The expression on his face suggested that he might be about to throw up. I kept an eye on him. What was coming next would be hard to look at.

Earlier that morning, I'd stopped by the Medical ICU to see if they had any alcoholic patients. They're prime examples of portal hypertension, a condition that develops in patients with cirrhosis of the liver. (Korea, Vietnam and the Middle East have made our nation's VA hospitals a seemingly inexhaustible gold mine for medical school professors and researchers.) This day there were three alcoholic veterans to be studied. Two were being sedated to control delirium tremens. The third guy was bleeding internally.

Angus had a tough time climbing the two flights of stairs, but he made it to the Medical ICU. All the beds were occupied. Nurses were scurrying about caring for their critically ill patients and assisting the doctors.

The gastroenterology fellows and their attending physician were trying to endoscope a patient who had arrived from the ER with upper gastro-intestinal bleeding. The patient promptly vomited blood all over the ICU doctors, nurses and himself. A bag of blood was being pumped into the patient as fast as possible because his own blood – the color of dark port wine – was pouring out of his rectum.

The stench of blood and feces was overpowering. I saw Angus cover his mouth with his hands and rush to the bathroom. I figured my students had seen enough. We left the gastroenterologists to their bloody work and moved to the far end of the ICU.

The patient I wanted the students to see was sound asleep and snoring. An IV was running into his arm. His vital signs and oxygen saturation levels were being monitored electronically.

"This man came in last night suffering from DTs," I told the group. "He'd stopped drinking two days earlier. That allowed the DTs to strike. It began with tremors which continued through the onset of hallucinations. The patient began to see helicopters whirling around his room. He'd had this happen before and had enough sense to get himself to the hospital.

"They had to sedate him intravenously with almost 200 mg. of Valium over a period of several hours before they could calm him down. Now, as you can see, he's sleeping like a baby."

I moved them to another patient nearby. "This guy over here came in about the same time as the other guy, also with DTs. But he didn't need as much sedation to control the symptoms of alcohol withdrawal. He's awake and very calm now."

"Then why is he still here?" a student asked. "The ICU seems to be full-up. Don't they need an extra bed for really critical patients?"

"Because patients suffering from DTs need really close observation," I told him. "There aren't enough nurses on a regular ward to provide that kind of care. Patients going through alcohol withdrawal are completely unpredictable. A sleeping patient may suddenly wake up when the Valium wears off and he may need additional sedation immediately. If he doesn't get it, he could become violent and maybe harm himself or the nurses. So treating DT patients on a regular ward is a bad idea.

"IT'S DANGEROUS TO FORGET how serious DTs can be. In one case I know about, the patient didn't get enough sedation and wasn't observed closely enough. He jumped out of a fourth floor window. He survived, but he's a paraplegic. The state medical board criticized the hospital for not having enough nursing personnel on that ward."

The man in the bed showed absolutely no interest in the young strangers standing at his bedside or in anything we were discussing. He was calm, all right.

"In another case," I continued, "the patient was over-sedated and wasn't monitored closely. He died before anybody noticed that he had stopped breathing. And then there was the patient suffering from severe alcohol withdrawal who received almost no sedation at all. He died of uncontrolled DTs."

I glanced at the man in the bed and thought I detected a slight smile. Maybe, or maybe not. My students weren't smiling.

"Never," I went on, "never underestimate how life-threatening DTs can be. Never treat DTs on a regular ward. A patient suffering with DTs must be observed closely and never treated on an out-patient basis."

Angus reappeared, pale and gaunt.

"You can skip the rest of rounds if you don't feel up to it," I told him.

"No, I'll keep going," he said. "I feel better now." He sure didn't look better, but he did look determined not to quit. So we moved on to another patient.

"This man has a Blakemore tube in place. As you can see, he's jaundiced and his abdomen is distended. That's due to ascites, which is water in the abdomen secondary to cirrhosis. His muscle wasting is due to malnutrition and years of continuous drinking. The bruises on his body are due to inadequate clotting caused by severe liver disease. Notice the loss of body hair, also secondary to liver disease."

I leaned over and bent the patient's elbow, slightly pushing his wrist backward. At this point, his hand began to flap as if he were waving goodbye. "That's called a liver flap," I said as I motioned the students into the hall where the patient couldn't hear us discussing his case. The man was barely conscious, but you can never be sure how much a patient in that state can hear and understand – if anything.

"That man's kidneys are beginning to fail," I said quietly, once we were out of earshot. "His liver is beginning to fail also. That's what the liver flap tells you. It's a very serious sign. It's usually a signal of the liver's final failure. The patient isn't likely to survive more than a few days."

"There's no way to save him?" Angus asked.

"He's too far gone," I said. "He certainly couldn't tolerate a major operation like a porta-caval shunt."

Before I could elaborate, there was a loud shout from the ICU.

"Get that God damn tube away from me!"

"Stay here," I told my students. I went inside to find out what the problem was.

The gastroenterologists were having trouble with a patient who had just been brought up from the ER. "Massive bleeding from esophageal varices and he won't let us use the Blakemore. He's refusing it." The young doctors were breathing hard from the physical exertion it took to deal with this man.

"Let me talk to him," I said. "What's his name?"

"Robinson. Jake Robinson."

The man in the bed glared at me as I approached and promptly vomited a huge amount of blood and blood clots. A quick-thinking nurse managed to catch most of the vomit in a basin.

"OK, Jake," I said. "Listen up! Your drinking's finally caught up with you! You are bleeding to death! You got that? You'll be dead in ten minutes if you don't let me put this tube in your nose and stick it down your throat! Cold stone dead in ten minutes! And that's the truth!" I kept my eyes locked on his.

"This tube here – it's got a balloon tucked inside it. If we can get it down inside your stomach, we can inflate the balloon. It will press against the place where the blood's coming from and stop the bleeding.

"You understand that? There's a damn good chance this tube will save your life! So, what's it going to be, Jake? You've got ten minutes!"

Jake's eyes were wide open now.

"Do you want to live or do you want to die today?"

"No, Sir," he whispered. "I surely don't."

"Then you *will* let me put this tube down your throat, right now. Is that right, Jake?"

"Yes, Sir," he said.

I asked the nurse to bring me a straw and a large coffee cup filled with ice and water. While I waited for her to return, I talked quietly to Jake, trying to lower his anxiety level as I lubricated the Blakemore tube with Vaseline.

The Blakemore is larger and certainly more intimidating than most tubes doctors push down nostrils. It has three air passageways, called lumens, two for balloons and one for sucking out liquid. I couldn't blame this battle-hardened veteran for staring at it in horror.

"It won't feel as bad as it looks," I told Jake. "The nurse is going to put a straw in your mouth. The straw goes into a cup of really cold ice water. When I tell you to start, I want you to suck the ice water up that straw and swallow – and keep on sucking and swallowing fast and hard!

"And don't quit! Keep sucking and swallowing fast and hard and we'll have this tube down in your belly in a flash. Are you ready, Jake?"

Jake reached for the sidebars of his bed and shut his eyes tight. His grip was so strong that his knuckles turned white.

"I'm ready," he said.

"Okay, Jake." I slowly inserted the tube into his nostril. "Don't do anything until this tube gets to the back of your nose. There! Suck! Swallow!

"Let's go for it, Jake. Suck! Swallow! Keep swallowing! Don't stop!

"You're doing great! Keep swallowing! And Stop!

"That's it, that's it! We're in, Jake! You did fine! Just fine! The tough part's over, so just try to relax and let the doctors do their job. The tube's in and it's going to save your life."

My students had been watching this whole scene. I joined them and gave them a play-by-play account of the procedure they were now observing.

"The GI team is putting 100 cc of air into the gastric balloon. They're pulling the tube back up so that the gastric balloon presses up against Jake's diaphragm. And now they're inflating the esophageal balloon to stop his bleeding.

"What's the third lumen for?" a student asked.

"It's for suctioning out the stomach below the balloons."

"What happens if this doesn't work, if they can't stop the bleeding?"

"In that case, they'll try again with a Linton tube which has a larger balloon. But it looks like that won't be necessary. So let's get out of here." I led them along the corridor to the stairs.

"How many times have you done that stuff with the Blakemore, Dr. Kessler?"

"I can't remember exactly. I've probably passed those tubes more than a hundred times. The key to success is the ice water. It inhibits the gag reflex. Remember that. And remember to wear your scrubs in the Medical ICU, never your street clothes. It can get to be a bloody mess."

AFTER LUNCH, I HELD my weekly conference with my third-year students. The subject, of course, was portal hypertension due to cirrhosis of the liver. I spent considerable time describing the various shunting procedures to divert blood away from a high-pressure system into the low-pressure systemic veins, such as the vena cava.

I talked about TIPS, the technique used by radiologists to create a shunt within the liver without having to resort to a major operation. I concluded the meeting by advising the students to refer alcoholic and drug addicted patients to colleagues who have a special interest and expertise in treating substance abuse.

"When we were up in the ICU, I told you about several cases of DTs where the haphazard use of tranquilizers led to unfortunate outcomes. When you become physicians, don't ever get involved with active alcoholics and drug addicts unless you have the knowledge to treat them. The same applies to those of you who will become surgeons.

"Don't ever try to perform the shunting procedures I've described unless you've had considerable training in that area of vascular surgery. Shunts are some of the most difficult surgical procedures done in the abdomen. So over-estimating your own competence can be a deadly mistake. The occasional practitioner – the surgeon short on training and experience – is likely to screw up, get into trouble and cause a lot of damage."

I told my students about a case I had reviewed involving a middle-aged man who underwent an H-graft shunt between the superior mesenteric vein and the vena cava. The surgeon didn't use portography, so he didn't have pre-operative X-rays of the veins in the patient's abdomen. He didn't measure the portal pressure before and after the procedure. He used a branch of the superior mesenteric vein that was too small.

And he placed two sump drains next to the synthetic graft. That allowed a retrograde passage of bacteria to infect the graft which clotted and became disconnected. It was clear to me that this surgeon lacked the experience to be doing this particular operation. The patient, by the way, bled to death.

I told the students about another surgeon who attempted to do a distal spleno-renal shunt. He tied off the wrong end of the splenic vein. This patient also bled to death, this time from the esophageal varices.

"Did those surgeons get sued?" a student asked.

"Yes, indeed," I said as I gathered up my papers. "And both cases were settled out of court. But that's not exactly the point I'm trying to make. Getting sued is an unpleasant experience, to be sure. However, it doesn't compare to getting dead. So I want you guys to remember not to take on cases that you haven't been trained to handle properly. Put the patient in the hands of someone who really knows what to do. See you all next week."

ALL THE STUDENTS LEFT the conference room except Angus who still looked a little green around the gills. I asked him if he was feeling any better.

"Lunch helped," he said. "But I wanted to ask you something, Dr. Kessler. How many alcoholics do you think you've treated over the years?"

"Thousands," I told him. "Literally, thousands."

"Wow, thousands. That's a lot." He paused a moment before plunging ahead.

"How can you tell if someone's an alcoholic? I have a friend who thinks he might be, but he doesn't know what to do about it and I don't know what to tell him."

"I can give you some suggestions, Angus. Let's go to my office and talk about it. What did you think of this morning's rounds?"

"Well, I didn't see everything, but what I saw was pretty awful. Was that guy really going to be dead in ten minutes if you didn't get that tube down his nose?"

"I might have been off by a minute or two. I've seen some guys in his condition bleed out and die in just five minutes. It can happen that fast. But we got the job done, once he understood the reality of his situation."

"What are his chances now?"

"Not good. He may squeak through this crisis physically, but he's still an alcoholic and his denial system is still intact. You've seen how strong it is. He wasn't able to grasp that his life was hanging by a thread, not until I got tough with him. Even if he survives and walks out of here, he'll tell himself he had a bit of bad luck, a bad accident, just one of those things that happen, not a signal to stop drinking.

"Denial is powerful and deadly, Angus. His alcoholism won't allow him to make the connection between the boozing and the hemorrhaging. And that's going to kill him. Sooner or later; probably sooner."

I settled myself behind my desk and told Angus to take a seat and relax. "To answer your question about diagnosing alcoholism: I'd say it exists when the consumption of alcohol causes a problem that screws up a person's life."

"What kind of problem?"

"Could be any kind of problem: health problem, work problem, relationship problem or a problem with the law, like getting arrested for driving while intoxicated."

"Why would getting a DWI indicate alcoholism? Lots of people get those."

"Really?" I said. "Well, I suppose a teenager getting drunk for the first time and getting a DWI might not mean much of anything. But if it keeps happening, it's probably pathognomonic of alcoholism."

"Patho…what?"

"Pathognomonic means that something is absolutely diagnostic of something."

Angus thought about that for a minute and then switched gears. "I've heard that AA can help alcoholics control their drinking. Is that right?"

"No, that's wrong." I said. "Alcoholics, by definition, are unable to control their drinking, not for any length of time. Alcoholism is a progressive disease. It can't be cured, only arrested. An alcoholic might be able to go on the wagon for a while, but the disease doesn't go away.

"If the alcoholic ingests alcohol, for whatever reason, the disease is activated and the progression resumes – not from where it began but from where it left off. AA can help an alcoholic stop drinking and stay stopped. But it can't transform an alcoholic into a moderate or so-called social drinker. No more than you can turn a pickle back into a cucumber."

"So that means not drinking at all forever, I guess," said Angus. "I don't think my friend could handle that."

"Maybe not, but a lot of people have been able to. Your friend should at least check it out."

I reached into my desk drawer and took out one of the booklets I kept there. "Here's something you can give your friend. It lists over 1,500 AA meetings in the Greater New York City area by day, time and location.

"You'll see some have an 'O' designation. That means they're open to non-alcoholics, so you could take your friend to one. He could listen to some recovering alcoholics tell how they got sober and stayed sober. He'll hear some damn good drinking and recovery stories.

"And if you go to more than one meeting with him, you'll learn more about alcoholism than you'll ever learn in most medical schools. So, I'll see you tomorrow, Angus," I said as he left my office. "I sure hope this helps your friend."

In the weeks that followed our conversation, I noticed that Angus started to look healthier. He become more attentive and involved. He went on to graduate from medical school and embarked on his career as a physician.

That was several years ago. From what I hear on the grapevine, Angus and his imaginary friend are still going to AA meetings and staying sober. That's good news. What this country doesn't need is one more impaired physician.

22

THE IMPAIRED PHYSICIAN

NOT ALL ALCOHOLICS ARE denizens of Skid Row. I'd wager that more alcoholics live in split-levels, mansions and penthouses than on the street. Alcoholics tend to function pretty well on the job, sometimes brilliantly, and tend to look down on "amateurs" who get roaring drunk once or twice a year on special occasions such as St. Patrick's Day, the office Christmas party, or your daughter's wedding.

Alcoholics tend to be clever about concealing the extent of their drinking, at least until the progression of their disease inevitably accelerates. Good performance helps an alcoholic to escape detection for years. That's why colleagues, as well the general public, are so shocked when a respected politician, religious leader or medical professional winds up on the front page of a tabloid newspaper.

Most people have a remarkable ability to ignore, overlook or even deny the obvious – until it's too late to help. I recall reading an article that said the last thing to go in an alcoholic's life was the job. It also made the point that less than 25% of alcoholic physicians had ever been confronted by an employer or medical society.

That's not surprising to me because many medical professionals – like most other Americans – think that doctors are immune or exempt from this disease. Unfortunately, they are not. And these impaired physicians are in a position to do much more harm than the run-of-the-mill drunk.

Consider this case that I was once asked to review. It involved a 66-year-old female who was admitted to the hospital with a 12-hour history of cramping abdominal pain in the upper quadrants. The admitting diagnosis was pancreatitis. A subsequent CT scan ruled this out. An ultrasound revealed dilated loops of small bowel; that's indicative of a bowel obstruction. Demerol was given to alleviate the pain.

By the third hospital day, the patient became distended and started to vomit. She was getting IVs and being fed a soft diet. Her vomiting was treated with Compazine which is contraindicated in patients with bowel obstruction.

The following day, she was even more distended and her abdomen was tender. She was fed orange juice and eggs which she promptly regurgitated. The doctor was called and he ordered more Compazine and Demerol. She was also getting a sleeping pill. On the fifth hospital day, she still had abdominal pain and again was treated with Demerol. The nurses' notes said that "the doctor does not want a naso-gastric tube."

On the sixth hospital day, the doctor ordered Milk of Magnesia because the patient had not yet had a bowel movement (Laxatives in the presence of obstruction may cause a perforation.) On the seventh hospital day, the woman's abdomen was firm and continued to be distended. She continued to receive Demerol and Compazine.

By 1:30 p.m., she developed chest pain, rapid respiration (35), a pulse of 140. Her lips were blue. By 3 p.m., her abdomen was large, firm, tympanitic and tender. At 5:30 p.m., she was given a full liquid diet. Her skin was clammy. By 8:30 p.m., she was sweating, short of breath and her blood pressure was down to 92/68. By 9:30 p.m., her skin was pale and her blood pressure was down to 84. At 10 p.m., a surgeon was finally called to see this patient. He found her in a state of shock and had her taken to the OR.

Exploration of the woman's abdomen revealed adhesions caused by a previous surgery. It was this scar tissue, which caused the bowel obstruction, which, in turn, caused gangrene of a segment of the bowel. The gangrenous bowel was removed and continuity restored with an end-to-end anasthemosis. The patient went on to develop multiple organ failure and died of sepsis one month later.

That case never went to trial. It was settled out of court. But I was prepared to recommend that the doctor be sued for:

1) Clouding the symptoms and physical findings with narcotics, sedatives and anti-emetics in a case of undiagnosed abdominal pain;

2) Not using a Levin tube in a patient who was vomiting;

3) Feeding a patient who was vomiting;

4) Failure to get a surgical consult by Day Two; and

5) Giving a laxative to a patient with a bowel obstruction.

Over the years, I reviewed numerous cases in which the bad outcome was the direct result of the same five deviations listed above. As far as I know, none of the doctors involved in those cases was impaired, just incompetent. In this case, I had been unable to connect the negligence with any substance abuse but, given what I learned later, it probably was a factor.

The doctor, I learned, had been sued before and – after this case was settled – he was removed from the staff of his hospital. He was later treated for substance abuse in a rehabilitation facility. But at the time I reviewed his case, I had no idea of how far along the road to rehab the doctor had progressed. Nor, I suppose, had his colleagues and patients.

IT'S REASONABLE TO ASSUME that the abuse of alcohol and other drugs by a doctor must have an adverse effect on the quality of medical care. The connection is obvious when a drunken obstetrician botches up a delivery and the result is a brain-damaged baby. (A jury award of $9-million in such a case, though rare, is not excessive, considering the care the child will need as long as he or she lives.)

The connection is less obvious when the deviations from accepted medical procedures consist of procrastination, masking of symptoms with drugs, and failure to obtain timely consultation.

Medical treatment rendered by impaired physicians is rife with bizarre consequences directly caused by their substance abuse. For example: a surgeon makes rounds and ignores his most recent patient. He has no recollection of the appendectomy he performed on the patient the night before. He had operated successfully in an alcoholic blackout.

Nobody died; nobody got sued. But that's not the point. It happened. If his colleagues were aware of his performing surgery in a blackout, they did nothing about it. I'd call that protecting the doctor, not his patients.

Several years ago, I reviewed a case for a law firm where a surgeon performed an umbilical hernia repair. Trouble was: the hernia wasn't there. Another surgeon had to perform a second operation to repair what the first surgeon missed: a large hernia *above* the patient's belly button.

Later, the patient recalled smelling alcohol on the first surgeon's breath just before his first operation and wished he had said something. What should he have done? Patients who detect alcohol on the breath of their physician during hospital rounds or office visits need to find another doctor. That's hard to do when you've been sedated and wheeled into the operating room.

But what about nurses, technicians, administrators and other doctors? If they become aware that a doctor on hospital duty has tremor, slurred speech or "boozy" breath, they should sound the alarm that this physician has a problem that cries out for immediate treatment. That takes a lot of courage.

Colleagues need to intervene and force the doctor into treatment. The intervention should involve family, fellow doctors, administrators and professionals who have the skill to break through the denial that impaired physicians have erected to protect their drinking or drug abuse. Throughout the nation, there are programs that can help the medical profession deal with this problem and treat health care professionals who want to salvage their right to practice medicine.

The existence and misguided protection of impaired physicians is a persistent problem that the medical community historically has ignored or attempted to sweep under the rug. Fortunately, progress has been made in chipping away that wall of silence and giving patients the facts they need to protect themselves.

But continuing to accept the myth of "frivolous lawsuits" or denying that real problems really exist does seem to conflict with the oath physicians make "to do no harm." Denial, collective as well as individual, inevitably leads to disaster.

HOW STRONG IS DENIAL? Consider the physician, an anesthesiologist, who failed to show up for work for a couple of days in a row and didn't answer repeated phone calls to his apartment.

Worried colleagues went to his home and found him in cardiac arrest. He was sprawled in the foyer with an IV bottle hanging on a coat rack. The IV line led directly into a vein in his arm. The IV bottle contained Fentanyl, a synthetic narcotic that anesthesiologists use in their work.

He was rushed to the hospital where he remained critically ill for several days, his breathing dependent on a respirator and his body monitored by the sophisticated devices in the ICU.

When he awoke from his self-induced coma, he was confronted by a psychiatrist who informed him that he would be transferred to the floor that treats drug addicts.

"I am shocked and insulted," he told the psychiatrist in icy tones: "This certainly does not apply to me. I am only a recreational user."

The anesthesiologist's colleagues did the right thing by getting him into treatment. Had they chosen to cover up the incident and minimize its significance, they would have become what trained clinicians call "enablers."

Enablers also suffer from denial and they also need help. And, yes, there are treatment programs for them, too.

23

CRACKING "THE CODE OF SILENCE"

M Y DOCTOR FRIEND ARNIE was a radiologist at the VA hospital and we had worked together for almost 30 years. "What's it like to testify against another doctor, Dick? I've always had mixed feelings about that."

Arnie had been asked to review some X-rays for a law firm representing a patient who was suing her doctors for medical malpractice. But before agreeing to participate, he wanted to research the subject of expert testimony and its use in potential medical liability cases. Arnie knew I'd done consulting work for law firms and insurance companies, so he called me for advice. I knew what he was going through because I'd gone through it myself, many years before.

Like every other kid in my grammar school, I'd learned that "nobody likes a tattle-tale" and I shared the belief that it was dishonorable to "snitch." By and large, schoolboys of my days were as tight-lipped about a classmate's questionable activities as members of the Mafia. It's hard to go against that childhood code of honor as we grow up.

Today's gangsters, I gather from the newspapers, seem willing to ignore the age-old tradition of *Omerta* and implicate their buddies, if it suits their own purposes. It's much harder for us honest folk – cops, bishops and doctors, for example – to break the laws of childhood and "rat out" our guilty friends and colleagues.

I knew that Arnie wanted to do the right thing, but dreaded feeling like a disloyal "tattletale." So I was glad to help him out. "Most of what I can tell you is based on my own experience," I said. "So I'll dig up some reliable reference material to back up my opinions. Let's meet tomorrow for lunch at the medical school."

That evening, I rummaged through my files to find some medical journal articles that contained official statements about doctors acting as medical expert witnesses. It took me some time to find what I was looking for because my filing system is what I choose to call idiosyncratic rather than haphazard.

Sure enough, the very last reference I found was the most important: a statement on "the physician acting as an expert witness," published in the Bulletin of the American College of Surgeons and revised periodically by the College's Judiciary Committee.

I selected the most recent statement from the August, 2008 issue. It was the first thing I asked Arnie to read when I had lunch with him the next day.

"*Physicians understand that they have an obligation to testify in court as expert witnesses on behalf of the plaintiff or defendant as appropriate. The Physician who acts as an expert witness is one of the most important Figures in malpractice litigation. Physician expert witnesses are expected to be impartial and should not adopt a position as an advocate or partisan in the legal proceedings . . . Compensation of the physician expert witness should be reasonable and commensurate with the time and effort given to preparing for deposition and court appearance . . . the physician expert witness is ethically and legally obligated to tell the truth.*"

"That's clear enough," said Arnie when he finished reading the abstract. "But I've never been asked to do this before. It still makes me a little uncomfortable."

"I felt the same way when I began reviewing cases for lawyers, Arnie. But I found that, more times than not, my evaluations were helpful to the doctor or hospital being challenged. I'd review about a dozen cases each year and 60% of the time I found no evidence of negligence. That saved the doctors, hospitals and attorneys a lot of time and money because I was able to advise the lawyers that they had no case and that they should forget about taking any legal action."

"I guess that's something lawyers don't want to hear."

"On the contrary. Good lawyers want to know right away if they don't have a valid case of negligence that will hold up in court. They don't want to put their money into a case they probably can't win. That would cost them $30,000 on average."

"Why would losing cost so much?"

"Because they have to pay for everything up front. They pay for copies of X-rays and all medical records. That cost can be considerable. They pay fees to expert witnesses, plus travel expenses if the experts testify at deposition or trial. It can really add up, especially if several different experts are used in a single trial. For example, a radiologist, a surgeon and an internist.

"The costs can be astronomical if the expert takes advantage of the system. I know of a patient's lawyer who couldn't afford to use a top-notch neurosurgeon because he requested a flat fee of $50,000 to review a case and testify."

"That's a ridiculously high fee!" said Arnie. "But isn't it possible that he set his fee that high so that lawyers would stop bothering him?"

"That could be, I guess. I'm not a mind reader. But take a look at this article from the *Journal of the American College of Surgeons*. 'Honesty Is the Only Policy: Physician Expert Witnesses in the 21st Century.' It says that physician experts in 2002 were being paid $300 to $800 per hour – and even more."

"That's a lot less than 50 Grand," said Arnie. "But it's still a lot of money."

"I think so, too. Take a look at that paragraph."

"Wow!" said Arnie. "This guy made $220,000 a year as an expert witness! Makes you wonder about conflict of interest, doesn't it?" He leaned back in his chair and took a deep breath. "Can I ask what kind of fees you charged, Dick?"

"Sure you can. I started at $50 an hour in 1970 and ended up at $200 an hour in 2005. My fees for malpractice consultations accounted for only about five percent of my annual income. I also did a lot of consultations for nothing."

"You're kidding,"

"No, I'm not. Over a 35-year period, I got about 2,000 phone calls from lawyers and law firms. I'd discuss the basics of the case for a few minutes and 90% of the time I'd be able to tell them right away that their case wasn't worth pursuing. I never billed for those phone conversations – except for one time when the call lasted well over an hour because the attorney couldn't take 'no' for an answer."

"Have you ever reviewed cases for the defense or testified in court on behalf of the doctor?"

"Oh sure," I answered, "Most expert witnesses have done consulting for both plaintiffs and defendants. Not at the same time, of course. I'd say that about 20% of all the cases I reviewed were for defendants. But I actually testified at trial for the defense only once."

"Who pays you when you work for the defense?"

"The insurance company that provides the doctor's malpractice coverage foots the bill."

"How do lawyers find doctors who are willing to review medical records?"

"There are a lot of legal firms that defend doctors and hospitals that are being sued. And it's pretty easy for them to find an expert witness. They just look through their Rolodex and pick out a doctor they've used before.

"Also, thousands of doctors place ads in law journals saying that they're available to review potential malpractice cases. I've never done that myself because I never wanted to make a career out of reviewing cases. A dozen cases a year was all that I could handle. I got my cases through word of mouth, one lawyer recommending me to another."

"How often have you had to testify at a trial as an expert witness?"

"Very seldom. About once a year. In the cases where I've found evidence of a serious negligence, most were settled out of court. It saves everyone a lot of trouble and money to settle if that's going to be the probable outcome.

"You know, Arnie, not every physician who gets sued is a bad doctor. Many cases get dropped because they don't have merit to begin with. Some of our best doctors get sued because, being human, they make a mistake that causes harm. Generally, these doctors belong to a group of physicians who are more candid with their patients. They admit their mistakes and make every attempt to correct them.

"It's the repeat offenders that are the greatest problem. Doctors who've been sued multiple times need to take a long look at their deficient skills and take some action to improve. Or they should just retire from the practice of medicine.

"And doctors should also take a hard look at their bedside manners. Some patients seek out an attorney when the outcome of their medical treatment is less than they expected. Often, patients decide to take legal action because they feel that the physician was arrogant or had a bad attitude.

"I remember one former resident of mine who'd been sued multiple times. He was bright and competent, but his bedside manner was plain awful. He was completely devoid of empathy and didn't have a scintilla of sensitivity. That's not malpractice by any means. But he could have avoided a lot of legal headaches if he'd just learned how to smile at his patients or, at least, not be unpleasant."

"Suppose you review a case and you don't find evidence of malpractice. Do you get paid for your time?"

"Of course. Expert witnesses should get paid for their time regardless of the outcome. Otherwise, witnesses might tend to be biased. Unfortunately, too many are biased as it is and tend to stretch the truth.

"I'm aware of numerous cases where an expert has made false statements to help defend a colleague. I'm sure that experts for the patient have made false statements to bolster their criticism of a doctor's conduct. As for myself, I've always relied on the truth. That's what an expert is supposed to do."

"Do the courts ever appoint an expert to review a case?"

"The courts have the power to do that, I suppose, but I've never heard of a case where that's happened. I doubt that the courts would pay enough to attract medical experts."

After a long silence, Arnie began asking about the attitude of the medical profession towards doctors who testify against other doctors.

"Can the medical societies or university department heads bring pressure to bear to discourage testifying on behalf of a patient?"

"They can and sometimes they do."

"Have you ever been discouraged from doing consultations for a patient?"

"Oh, yeah. But before I get into that, let me show you another article. The June, 2000, *Bulletin of the American College of Surgeons* states their policy:

'No organization should attempt to interfere with or seek to influence any member's legal right to testify or provide an opinion regarding a case (submitted for review). To do so would come close to witness tampering or interference.'

"Now I'm sure that every medical society and medical school in the United States would agree officially with that policy of non-interference with the honest testimony of expert witnesses. But let me tell you about my experience.

"After I'd testified at my very first trial, which was held in Chicago, one member of the defense firm representing the physicians contacted the Veterans Administration in Washington to complain that a full-time physician with the VA was moonlighting, doing medical legal work and being paid for it."

"Well, that's ridiculous," Arnie, said. "We're allowed to do legal consultations, as long as we do it on our own time. At least, that's what I've been told."

"You're correct," I assured him. "And the lawyer was informed of that fact by the VA. And he was reprimanded by a judge in Chicago for trying to interfere with expert witness testimony."

"That's good to know," said Arnie.

"Lawyers tell me that the VA is an excellent source of expert witnesses because we don't have private practices that could be threatened. If you're in private practice, your livelihood often depends on referrals from other doctors. So, if you're testifying for patients or their families, you run the risk of having those referrals cut off. That's especially true in small towns and small cities."

"Well, that's not good, but it's understandable."

"Yeah, it is. But that's why lawyers for the plaintiff have a hard time finding experts who will testify against a doctor in their own community or hospital. The attorneys usually have to go out of town – and sometimes across the country – just to find a willing expert. Of course, lawyers don't have any trouble finding physicians who'll testify for the defense of a local doctor or hospital."

"How about universities and medical schools? Wouldn't an academic position in an ivory tower give a doctor some protection from intimidation?"

"You'd think so, but I know of a doctor here in New York who was chief of surgery in a hospital affiliated with a medical school. The chairman of the department called him in and told him he didn't want him to testify for patients any more. But it would be OK to testify on behalf of doctors."

"What did the surgeon do?"

"He ignored it."

"So what happened to him?"

"Nothing," I said. "He figured that the chairman was bluffing. But a less confident doctor probably might have folded."

Since we were on this subject of intimidation, I showed Arnie a letter I got from a lawyer after I had testified in court for one of his clients.

"*Dear Doc,*" it started out. "*I am pleased to report to you that at the conclusion of the plaintiff's case, but I might add, not before that point in time, the defendants negotiated a settlement of this case. The plaintiff was most appreciative of your efforts on her behalf and has asked me to convey that to you. Once again, thanks for all your direction in this case, and I look forward to the opportunity when it next presents itself to work with you.*

"*In line with our conversation concerning the pressure put upon physicians by the organized Defense Bar and Insurance Companies, I have just within the last three days received word from Dr.——, of eminent national reputation of the —— School of Medicine who had reviewed an obstetrical case for me three years ago and had indicated in writing that, not only were there obvious record changes and gross departures from any standard of accepted medical care and that he would be happy to testify in this case. He has now indicated that he is being pressured not to appear any longer in plaintiff's cases, despite the merits and, accordingly, will not be able to assist us in this regard.*

"*I recall your comment that you did have a handle on an orthopedist and perhaps an OB/GYN specialist who might be available on such matters and, if that be so, I would genuinely appreciate some identification of them . . . . Please feel free to give me a call.*"

ARNIE SLID THE LETTER back across the table. "So even the best medical schools in the country intimidate doctors," he said. "Even when they say they don't."

"Yeah, and that kind of pressure is harder to deal with than an actual threat, like the one I received some years ago.

"I was getting ready to fly to Texas to testify for a plaintiff in a medical malpractice case. I got a greeting card with a picture of a cowboy on his horse. Inside the card was a typed note: *'JFK was told to stay out of Texas. He didn't listen and look what happened to him.'* Of course, there was no return address and no signature.

"The judge hearing this case wouldn't let the card to be read or shown to the jury because it was too inflammatory. I guess the judge exhibited good judgment. My getting a threatening anonymous mail really had no bearing on the merits of the case."

"I agree," said Arnie. "But intimidation by some unknown individual has to be frightening."

"Yeah, it is. But I've found that most threats are just empty words from angry people who can't back them up with action. What's really tough to deal with is what I call 'institutionalized intimidation' by misguided colleagues, professional groups, and institutions that throw real sticks and real stones that can do you serious damage. That's something else to think about.

"Remember during the early years of laparoscopic surgery? There were a lot of bile duct injuries because of the lack of experience of the surgeons performing them. To learn how to do laparoscopic removal of the gall bladder, they'd take a weekend course where they would 'see one, do one, and teach one.' Well, as you can imagine, attorneys during the early 90's were kept busy suing surgeons who had damaged bile ducts without recognizing their mistake.

"Several of those laparoscopic cholecystectomy cases were referred to me for review. I had limited experience with this new type of surgery myself, so I referred the attorneys to a couple of surgeons in West Virginia who were not only familiar with the technique but also taught the method to other surgeons.

"For a while, they were inundated with work, reviewing cases and testifying on behalf of patients whose bile ducts had been damaged by a surgeon's blunder. These two physicians later joined a surgical group in Ohio that wouldn't permit them to testify for patients. So a valuable source for honest appraisal quietly dried up.

"Prosecutors complain about the 'conspiracy of silence' in criminal cases. People who probably witnessed the crime are afraid to testify or just don't want to get involved. So they insist that they didn't see or hear anything. And neither does anyone else in the neighborhood. That makes it easier for guilty suspects to thwart an investigation and even avoid a trial. It's also a problem in civil cases, including medical malpractice cases."

"You're not talking about some organized conspiracy, are you?"

"No, not in the legal sense. It's more like the force of a prevailing opinion within a group – any group. Loyalty to the group demands that you resist any perceived attack or criticism that threatens an individual within your group, even if you think the individual is probably guilty of every charge the 'outsiders' are making.

"You tell yourself that the outsiders are just trying to give the profession a bad name – or the institution, or the church, or the town, or the neighborhood or whatever. So, if you're members of that group, you have to help circle the wagons. Stick together and keep your lips zipped.

"If you keep stonewalling long enough maybe the outsiders will give up and go away. If they don't, you start yelling at them, calling them bad names and battering them with propaganda. Whatever you do, you don't tell the truth."

"You're really pissed off, aren't you?" said Arnie. "But you're probably right. Driving into work, I hear a lot of talk about a malpractice crisis in this country: off-the-wall jury awards, skyrocketing malpractice insurance premiums, doctors forced to limit their practice, retire early or move to a different state."

"I hear the same stuff, too," I told him. "And I know some excellent doctors who've swallowed that guff hook, line and sinker.

"But I've read some reports by doctors and lawyers that suggest there's no cause-and-effect relationship between claims paid by insurance companies and the premiums they charge doctors."

"Some reporters should look into that, don't you think?"

"Shouldn't be too hard to find out," I said. "While they're at it, they should check the accuracy of an article I read by a lawyer who's represented doctor defendants as well as patient plaintiffs. According to him, the number of malpractice claims filed and the amount of jury awards has remained fairly stable. However, during that same period, malpractice premiums have gone through the roof."

"Why doesn't that surprise me?" said Arnie.

"Yeah, just like dogs. They do it because they can." I checked my watch. "Time for me to get to the anatomy lab, Arnie."

"Yeah," he said, "and I have to get back to the office and call the law firm that's been after me."

"Have you decided what you're going to tell them?"

"Well," said Arnie, "you got me thinking about 'do no harm.' Keeping silent, not getting involved, maintaining the *status quo*: that doesn't help anybody and it puts a lot of people in danger.

"So I think I'm going to tell the lawyers that I'll review their case and give them an honest opinion based on the facts. If it turns out that I have to testify, I guess I will."

24

THE FINAL NAIL
IN THE COFFIN

▬▬

IT WAS THE LAST TIME I would be meeting with this group
of third-year medical students. Their 12-week surgical rotation
was coming to an end. I was presenting a case of SOB – shortness
of breath – and the students were becoming more upset with
every word I uttered. It was clear to them that the 42-year-old
man I was telling them about was becoming the victim of blatant
incompetence and was not going to survive.

The man was one week post-op with a colon resection for
cancer. His clinical picture had been looking grim for several days.
His temperature, pulse and white blood count were elevated. His
abdomen was distended and silent. His pain was intensifying. He
was sweating profusely. He was pale and confused. One and a half
quarts of black liquid – old blood—had been sucked out of his
stomach. His urine output was low because of dehydration and
blood loss. His kidneys were beginning to fail.

"Completely disoriented, the man pulls out all of his tubes.
They are re-inserted. His respiratory rate now varies between
36 and 44 per minute. Why is he so confused, disoriented and
agitated?" I asked the class.

"Maybe he has delirium tremens from alcohol withdrawal,"
said a student. "Was he a heavy drinker?"

"He drank three-to-six beers every day. But that's not likely to
cause a significant alcohol withdrawal problem. This man has been
in the hospital for eight days and the symptoms of DTs usually
begin in the first 72 hours after cessation of drinking. So DTs are
a very unlikely cause of his confusion and disorientation. So why
is he delusional?"

"He's having a lot of trouble breathing," a bright student replied. "What were his blood gas measurements?"

"That's a very good question," I said. "The PO2 – oxygen – was 46."

"Wow! That's very low."

"Do you know how low oxygen affects the brain?"

"I know it can make the patient crazy and confused," a student responded. "Can it also make him agitated?"

"Absolutely," I said. "Patients with low oxygen are disoriented and difficult to control. They frequently get combative and pull out the various tubes going into their bodies."

"At this point in time," a student said, "what was his blood pressure?"

"The systolic pressure was 60."

"Then he's in shock. That can also have an adverse effect on the brain, can't it?"

"It sure can. Patients in shock are often irrational. What about the rapid respiration? He's breathing at a rate of 36-to-44 per minute. Is that a problem?"

"It's a big problem," a usually quiet student said. "At that rate, his respiratory muscles will fatigue eventually and his breathing will cease."

"I can see you've been reading about respiratory failure," I said. "So, how do you manage a patient like this?"

"Wouldn't you insert a tube into his windpipe?"

"Intubate him?" I said. "Yes, you would."

"And put him on a respirator?" the student continued.

"Absolutely. And all this has to be done before a patient stops breathing. Now let me ask you this: would you want to give the patient some sedation to counteract the agitation and bizarre behavior?"

"Well, sure," a student replied. "I guess you'd have to."

"When would you do that?"

"Anytime the patient is uncooperative."

"Wrong! Dead wrong! Never sedate an agitated patient until you know what's causing the agitation! That's important to remember.

"You see, if the behavior is due to brain hypoxia – low oxygen – even a small amount of narcotic or sedation may be the *coup de grace* that will stop the patient's breathing. That's especially true if a patient has been breathing very rapidly. And you should never, *never* sedate patients until you are ready to intubate them."

I paused to look at my notes. "Now let me tell you how this man's doctors actually managed his problem. They did *not* intubate him. They diagnosed DTs and began to give him Sparine and Valium."

"I can see what's coming," said a young woman. "I mean, the man had been bleeding! What was his hemoglobin?"

"Seven-point-six," I replied.

"Did they transfuse him?"

"No, they did not."

"That's terrible," she said. "Just terrible."

"Yes, it is." I looked around the conference table. "Who can tell me what might be causing all of this man's problems? Anyone have a diagnosis?"

"It sounds like septic shock from generalized peritonitis," a young man said.

"You're correct, but why the low oxygen?"

"Fluid in the lungs from shock due to sepsis."

"Right on!"

Another student asked, "Did they do a paracentesis?"

"Yes, they finally did a paracentesis and it showed intestinal contents in the abdominal cavity. Can anyone tell me why?"

"The intestinal suture line was leaking," another young woman said. "Is that what they found when they operated?"

"Well, before the surgeon could operate again, some idiot gave the poor patient 20 mg of Valium for delirium. The man had a respiratory arrest within the hour and could not be resuscitated. End of story."

"And they never intubated the patient?" the young woman said.

"Not until after the respiratory arrest."

"What did the autopsy show?"

"A major breakdown of the intestinal suture line."

The young woman who called it correctly said nothing. She just sat there, shaking her head. I waited for a minute or two.

There was a simple message I wanted these students to take away from this conference and remember for the rest of their lives: "Do not be the one to deliver the *coup de grace* or place the final nail in someone's coffin by sedating an agitated patient who is having difficulty breathing."

REPETITION'S A GOOD TEACHING tool. So I presented two more cases that illustrated how a physician's ignorance can cause a patient's death.

The first case concerned a 44-year-old woman who was hospitalized because of a flare-up of Chron's disease – a chronic inflammation of the bowel. She was kept in the hospital for one month while the staff tried to improve her nutritional status. This medical regimen did not improve her condition and so she was scheduled for surgery.

The woman's pre-operative tests revealed that she was suffering from pneumonia and an albumin of 2.0, which is quite low. She was taken to the OR for resectioning of her diseased large bowel. Immediately following surgery, she began to have trouble breathing. Her respirations were rapid (28-to-42) and her pulse went as high as 160.

One day after her operation, a chest X-ray revealed bilateral pneumonia. The tests of her blood gases revealed low oxygen and elevated CO_2. Her blood pressure was low and needed support with Dopamine. Her temperature soon rose to 103°.

Her doctors ordered a gallium scan to look for an abscess in her lungs or in her abdomen. But, on the morning of that scheduled test, the woman became very restless and confused. She was given morphine. Two hours later, because of her continued agitation, the woman was seen by a doctor who noted that her respirations were

40 per minute. He gave the woman eight milligrams of morphine and obtained a sample of blood for blood gas determination.

Unfortunately, no one waited for the results of the blood gas test. They turned out to be PO_2 12, PCO_2 59 and pH 7.20 which showed that the woman was almost dead from lack of oxygen and CO_2 retention.

But no one had seen this data before she was placed on a stretcher and taken to the radioisotope lab for the gallium scan. A few minutes later, she stopped breathing. She was resuscitated, but she had suffered severe brain damage. She died of pneumonia three weeks later.

THE LAST CASE I PRESENTED to the students that day was that of a 63-year-old man who had been admitted to the hospital for elective repair of a large incisional hernia. He had a history of smoking four packs of cigarettes daily for many years and he was known to have significant emphysema.

At 9:30 a.m. on the day of his surgery, his blood gases were measured. His pH, PCO_2 and HCO_3 were normal, but the tests revealed a PO_2 of 64 and an oxygen saturation of 90% – both very low. The man's surgery began at 11 a.m. and ended three-and-a-half hours later.

"Wait! Hold on!" Several students interrupted me before I could continue this presentation. "You mean they performed an elective operation on someone in that condition?"

They were all talking at once. "Please, Dr. Kessler!" one student said. "I can't take another horror story!"

"Aw, come on," said Ira the Mumbler. "I need to find out what happens. I'm applying to law school tomorrow."

Once again, the Mumbler had broken the tension.

"Before you start studying for the bar, Ira, perhaps you could tell us what the surgeon should have done."

"He should have cancelled the surgery!"

Another student jumped in. "He should have gotten a pulmonary consultation,"

"Or at least done some pulmonary function tests," said another.

"Those are all good suggestions," I told them. "Too bad nobody made them at that hospital. Anyhow, while the man was in the recovery room following his surgery, his blood gases were checked. The test showed that he had a pH of 7.25 – that's low – and a PCO_2 59 – that's high. He had a PO_2 97 and oxygen saturation of 93%. Now, what does all that mean?"

Hands shot up at once. I was pleased to see that my students had become very knowledgeable about blood gases. I called on a student sitting at the end of the table who said, "He's having trouble blowing off the CO_2 because of his emphysema."

"You're correct. How do you want to monitor his pulmonary function?"

"I'd get blood gas measurements several times a day."

"Right, again," I said. "But for the next three days, the man was monitored with a pulse oxymeter. Do you think that's okay?"

"No, I don't," he said without hesitation. "A pulse oxymeter only measures oxygen saturation. It doesn't tell you what's happening with the CO_2 or the pH."

"Correct," I said. "It's too bad you weren't managing this man's case. But you weren't. Over the next three days, his temperature went up to 103° and his respirations became rapid and labored at 36 per minute.

"At 4:00 a.m. of the fourth post-operative day, the nurses on duty saw that the man was restless and short of breath. They called the house doctor. Does anybody want to guess what he did?"

I could see that my students all dreaded what was coming.

"The house doctor administered the *coup de grace*," I said. "He gave the man Pantapon – a narcotic. And Vistaril – a sedative. Two hours later, the man stopped breathing altogether and could not be resuscitated."

I paused for a moment trying to decide if I needed to say anything more about the case. No, I thought, they all got the message: Don't drug a patient who's short of breath.

"WELL, LADIES AND GENTLEMEN," I said, "that concludes our last case and our last conference. I've enjoyed having you hang out with me here at the hospital for the past 12 weeks. You've been attentive, enthusiastic and hard-working. Quite frankly, I'll miss each and every one of you – even Ira. Good luck in your studies and keep up the good work. You should do just fine."

After all the other students gathered up their books and left the conference room, Ira approached me and asked, "What happened to the schmucks who took care of those patients you presented?"

"They all got sued, Ira. Successfully, I might add."

"Good! Serves them right!" He stuck out his hand. "Thanks, Dr. Kessler. Thanks a lot. For everything. It's been a great 12 weeks."

With that, Ira the Mumbler walked out of my life. I know that he graduated from NYU Medical School because I saw his name in the commencement program. But did he go on to law school after completing his medical studies? Or was he really just kidding? I have no idea. But I'm pretty sure that whatever career path he's on, Ira is doing no harm – and maybe a lot of good.

25

THE CADAVER ON TABLE 9

THE FIRST-YEAR STUDENTS were just about finished with their study of the human body. They had dissected the cadavers in the NYU Anatomy Lab from toe to thorax. Now only the head and neck regions remained to be fully examined. After that, I had told the students, they themselves would be examined – but not dissected.

The other two professors and I would spend an hour testing the knowledge of groups of eight-to-ten students assembled around a cadaver. There would be three sessions per day for two days. I arrived early that first morning to make sure all the cadavers still had intact those important structures we would be asking students to identify.

I had 26 cadavers to examine and I went from one body to the next, carefully exploring the neck dissections that had been done. I also checked the condition of the faces, which were exposed but only partially dissected.

I stopped before I got to the cadaver on Table 9. From the very beginning of the semester, I had been avoiding that particular one as much as possible.

I had known that my old friend and neighbor Joe had died, of course. I'd attended his memorial service. I remembered someone there telling me that Joe had willed his body to medical science, but I never gave it much thought. I certainly never expected that Joe would show up on a table in my anatomy laboratory.

Never before in all my years of teaching anatomy had I encountered the cadaver of a person I had known in life. But there he was on Table 9 when the semester began, another anonymous dead body shrouded by the white waterproof body bag with black trim.

Now, with the semester ending, I stood where I was, lost in thought. I'd check Joe's condition later.

WHEN I WAS A MEDICAL STUDENT, the study of anatomy was often boring – downright dull, in fact – even when the professor was a renowned anatomist like Dr. J.C.B. Grant. Students weren't shown the clinical applications of the anatomical structures that were staring them right in the face.

"What the hell do we need to know this for?" we'd ask each other. Or "Who gives a rat's ass about the nerve supply to the inferior gemellus muscle in the buttocks?"

We spent hours memorizing structures without knowing how this knowledge would apply when we finally became doctors. But anatomy courses today are using clinical examples of actual cases to stimulate students by demonstrating the importance of anatomy in a wide range of situations they may encounter as practicing physicians.

At New York University Medical School, Drs. Bruce Bogart and Vicky Harnik recently inserted 16 clinical case studies into the first-year anatomy course. Most are cases of common diseases that doctors see and treat frequently. Others are less common and some are actually rare syndromes that most doctors fail to recognize until it's too late for the patient.

It was pleasant to relish the evidence that sometimes things can change for the better. I checked my watch and congratulated myself on postponing my inspection of the cadaver on Table 9. I could do that later, after this final class ended.

IT WAS 10:00 A.M. The students were all present. They split up into three groups and gathered around their professors to discuss a case study concerning the thyroid gland. I asked my students to sign an attendance sheet and then ushered them to the rolling blackboard on which I had drawn a cross-section of a human neck at the level of the thyroid gland.

"Before we begin the case study," I said, "I want to introduce you to the signs and symptoms of a goiter which is defined as an enlargement of the thyroid gland." I pointed to a structure in the drawing. "What is this?"

"The trachea," they answered in unison.

"Commonly known as the windpipe because that's where our breath goes. And what's this structure behind the trachea?"

"The esophagus."

"Commonly known as the gullet because that's where our food goes. No one thinks that's funny? Then, let's move on. What's this tiny structure that runs in the groove between the trachea and the esophagus?" I waited for an answer.

"Nobody knows what this little dot is? Okay, let me spell it out for you." I picked up the chalk and labeled the little dot "recurrent laryngeal nerve."

"Oh, darn." I heard a young woman say. "How could I forget that?"

I turned around and picked her out. "Do you remember what that nerve does?"

"It innervates the muscles in the larynx that control the vocal cords."

"All the muscles?"

"All but one."

Which one?"

"The cricothyroid muscle."

"Very good." I looked around the circle and asked one of the young men. "Can you identify this structure wrapped around the front and sides of the trachea?"

"That's the thyroid gland."

"Correct. Now what sign or symptom would a person begin to notice if the thyroid gland enlarged outwardly?"

"A swelling in the front of the neck?"

"That's right, "I said. " So, for Number 1 on our list of signs and symptoms of goiters, let's write '*mass in the neck*' on the board. Tell me what could happen if the thyroid enlarged in the direction of the trachea and esophagus?"

"If it compressed the trachea," another student volunteered, "the person might have trouble breathing,"

"Absolutely. So, for Number 2, we'll put down *S.O.B.* which is also short for shortness of breath." That produced group laughter and a couple of groans. One of the students asked: "Could the goiter compress the esophagus?"

"Sure, it could. So Number 3 is *dysphagia* – trouble swallowing. Anything else?" I looked around at the blank faces. "Come on, now! What would happen if pressure was applied to this little dot between the trachea and esophagus? Anybody?"

"Oh, of course!" Several students had the answer. "If the gland pressed against the recurrent laryngeal nerve, the person would have a hoarse voice!"

"Absolutely. So Number 4 is '*hoarse voice*'. There you have the signs and symptoms of a goiter determined by the anatomical relationship of the thyroid's proximity to adjacent structures. And my point is?"

"Knowing anatomy can be very useful in clinical medicine;" the students chorused.

"Oh, have I made that point before?" I put down my piece of chalk and left the blackboard. "Let's go over to our cadaver," I said. "I'm going to take you through a thyroidectomy, step by step, and I'll be asking you to identify the various structures."

"Have you done many thyroidectomies?" a student asked.

"About 50," I replied. "Most of them when I was a resident."

The young men and women gathered around the table and I picked up my scalpel.

"Watch what happens," I said. "A horizontal incision about four-to-five inches long is made in the lower third of the neck. After the skin and fat has been cut, what's the next layer the surgeon encounters?"

"The platysma muscle," a student answered.

"Show it to me," I said, pointing to the neck.

"Is this it?"

"Yes, that's it. What's its nerve supply?"

"The facial nerve."

"Correct. The surgeon then dissects the skin and muscle flaps up to the Adam's apple and down to the sternum. Then he opens the next layer by a vertical midline incision. Does anyone know what that layer is called?"

"The investing layer of deep cervical fascia," the first student answered.

"Show me."

"I believe it's that layer."

"Correct. The surgeon then has to lift the strap-muscles off the thyroid gland. What are the names of those muscles?"

"Sternohyoid, omohyoid, sternothyroid and thyrohyoid," the next student replied.

"Show me."

He pointed out the first three, but couldn't find the thyrohyoid.

"Let me help you," I said. "It's that short muscle there. The surgeon never sees that muscle during a thyroidectomy. Okay, the next step is to get control of the middle thyroid vein which is easily torn if not tied off first. Show me the middle thyroid vein."

The next student, a young woman, looked confused. "I've never seen a middle thyroid vein," she said. Several other students said that they hadn't seen one either.

"That's because you tore the vein the other day before your manual told you to look for it." I said. "Not your fault. But remember this when you're in the operating room. If you ever tear the middle thyroid vein before you locate it and tie it off, there will be blood all over the damn place. And that's when accidents happen. While you're trying to get control of this stinking little vessel, nerves can be damaged inadvertently."

I told the young woman that the cadaver still had one middle thyroid vein intact. "It's on the left side," I said. "So find it for me."

She bent over the cadaver, lifted up the strap muscles, and exclaimed, "Oh, my God! Here it is! Just like in *Grant's Atlas!* Wow!"

The other students closed in around the cadaver. "Let me see it!" "Let me see it, too!" "Me, too!" They kept chattering until all of them got to see the little middle thyroid vein for the very first time.

"Be careful not to tear it," I said. "We may want to use this specimen during the exam you'll be taking. And, yes, that's a hint." There were grateful smiles all around the cadaver.

"Okay, the next step is to lift up the lobe and rotate it medially to identify an important structure between the trachea and the esophagus. What is that?"

"The recurrent laryngeal nerve."

"Show me."

"It's here – in the groove between the trachea and the esophagus."

"Correct. And what does it do, again?"

"It innervates all the intrinsic muscles in the larynx. All of them except the cricothyroid."

"Very good. And what will happen if a surgeon cuts this nerve?"

"He'll get sued," said a young man.

"You'd better believe it. There's no excuse for that kind of blunder in a virgin neck. That's a neck that's never been operated on, one that's free of scar tissue"

"Have you seen that happen?"

"I've known of several cases over the years."

"Did the patients all have a hoarse voice afterward?"

"Yes."

"What can be done for that?"

"Not much. Teflon injections into the vocal cords seem to help, sometimes," I said. "What else can get injured in this area besides this nerve?"

Nobody had an answer. So I pointed to the neck and asked one of the young men to show me the esophagus. The student lifted up the thyroid and dissected behind the trachea. "Here it is," he said.

"Now I want all of you to take a close look at the esophagus. This is a very soft structure and it should never be damaged during a thyroidectomy. With careful dissection, it needn't be. But I know of a case where a surgeon cut a hole in a woman's esophagus and also cut one of her recurrent laryngeal nerves. That was a truly disastrous case. Very disturbing."

The students looked up from the cadaver and gave me their full attention. "Do you have time to tell us about it, Dr. Kessler?" said a young woman, obviously hoping for a full "time out."

"Okay," I said. "Let's pause for a moment, only because this sort of thing is something you should know about. The case involved a housewife, 32 years old and the mother of four small children. She developed a lump in her neck which occasionally caused a choking sensation.

"Her doctor examined her and decided that the lump was in the woman's thyroid gland and needed to be removed because there was a possibility of cancer. He referred her to a surgeon who removed most of the thyroid gland including the lump.

"By the following day, the young woman was experiencing severe pain and swelling in her neck and chest area. Even her face and tongue were swollen. It was obvious that an overwhelming infection was taking place and she was returned to the operating room for re-exploration of the neck.

"The surgeon found a big hole in her esophagus. Contaminated saliva was leaking through that hole into her neck. That was causing a fulminating infection. There was necrotic tissue – dead tissue – and foul smelling pus, which had to be removed and drained.

"A pathologist examined the thyroid tissue that had been removed the previous day and found that a large piece of normal esophagus had also been removed and was attached to the thyroid specimen. What had happened?

"Well, while performing the thyroidectomy, the surgeon had accidentally removed a 1 ½ inch by ¾ inch piece of normal tissue from the left side of the esophagus. He sewed it up without even knowing what he had done."

"Oh, my God, that's awful," one of the students exclaimed.

"The esophagus, as we've just seen here in the lab, is a very soft structure. It doesn't hold sutures well. So it quickly broke down and leaked. Furthermore, that important nerve that controls the vocal cords, the recurrent laryngeal nerve we've been looking at this morning? That was also cut. So the woman's voice became hoarse.

"At this point, all the surgeon could do was go back in and establish drainage with a 'spit fistula' and insert a tube through her belly into her stomach – the procedure's called gastrostomy – for feeding purposes. The woman was sent home with a tube sticking out of her neck to drain saliva. The infection persisted, however, and she had to be readmitted two weeks later – this time to a larger, university hospital – for drainage of a neck abscess and insertion of a different kind of drainage tube.

"Three weeks later the woman was admitted again to have her neck drained once more. One month after that, she went back to the hospital, this time to have a new esophagus made so that she could eat. Here's how they did that. They removed a piece of her large intestine from her abdomen and placed it in her chest."

"O, Sweet Jesus!" whispered one of my students.

"They took the upper end of the piece of her large intestine and connected it to the upper part of her damaged esophagus. Then they connected the lower end to her stomach. This procedure is called a colon interposition and what you wind up with is never as good as a normal esophagus.

"Only God can make a good esophagus, guys; there is really no replacement.

"Now, take a closer look at our cadaver. Note the position of the structures below the neck. In order to make room for the hook-up in the woman's neck, they had to remove part of her clavical – the collarbone here – and part of her sternum, the chest plate.

"What happened? Within three weeks she had developed a stricture in the upper connection so that she was regurgitating her food. The doctors tried stretching the esophagus, but the woman continued to have trouble swallowing. That's a condition we call dysphagia.

"Two weeks later she needed another operation to enlarge the entrance into her chest. That meant that more of the clavicle and sternum had to be resected, along with part of the first and second ribs."

A student nudged the young man next to him and said, "Can you believe that?" The other student just shook his head.

"One month later," I went on, "the woman was hospitalized and had a Teflon injection into her paralyzed left vocal cord to relieve the hoarseness. That seemed to work very well. Within two months, she was back to be dilated.

"Ten months later, the Teflon injection procedure had to be repeated. Within a year, she had to undergo multiple dilations to allow her to swallow food." The students looked bewildered.

"You're wondering how she's doing today, aren't you?" I said. "Currently, I hear, she requires dilation of the narrowed bowel – under anesthesia – every three months. She has so much trouble swallowing food that she eats alone now rather than subject her family to the sounds of her belching and regurgitation.

"Shortly after eating, she gets abdominal cramps and diarrhea. That's characteristic of a dumping syndrome, which is caused by severing nerves to the stomach during colon interposition.

"She can't lay flat because of acid reflux in her reconstructed esophagus. She has significant chest pain when she uses her arms. That's because so much bone was removed from her upper chest area. Her anemia is a recurring problem. Sometimes she needs to insert a tube down her throat into the stomach for feedings.

"Overall, this woman has undergone over 90 procedures, ten of which were major operations. But there's really nothing that can be done for her now. All her disabilities are permanent."

"So there was a lawsuit?"

"You bet there was," I said. "The woman's quality of life had been impaired forever because of a technical blunder that should never have happened. Even an expert witness for the defense stated in his pretrial deposition that a high school kid or a dummy couldn't cut a hole like that in a normal esophagus. Even so, he tried his best to defend his former resident."

"How could he defend him?" asked one of the young women. "On what basis?"

"Well, the expert witness had 'impressive credentials,' as they say. He was the former chairman of a surgical department at a medical school, a member of the Society of Head and Neck Surgeons, a member of the American Thyroid Association, a surgeon who had done thousands of thyroid operations himself.

"He tried his best to defend his former resident by implying that there had to have been a congenital abnormality of the woman's esophagus to make it vulnerable to injury. He stated in his deposition that it was not possible to injure a normal esophagus because the esophagus is not near the thyroid and is never seen during thyroid surgery."

"That's bullshit!" The angry student pointed to the cadaver's neck. "It's right there! Right next to the thyroid gland!"

"Yes, that's where it is," I said. "But not in his deposition. Obviously, he was prepared to give erroneous information to the jury, but he never made it to the witness box. After the woman's lawyer put into evidence some anatomical pictures that clearly showed the thyroid gland touching the esophagus, the defense wisely decided not to put their expert witness on the stand."

"So he didn't get a chance to lie," said the angry student. "Did you testify in that trial, Dr. Kessler?"

"Yes, I did. I gave the jury pretty much the same anatomical information I gave to you just now."

"What happened?"

"The jury awarded the plaintiff two million dollars and that was upheld by the State Supreme Court."

"Thank God, she got a good verdict," a young woman said. "Is that surgeon still operating?"

"Last I heard, he was," I said. "Later, after this case was decided, he was sued for accidentally tying off a renal artery without knowing it. That patient lost a kidney. But the jury let the doctor off the hook because they were under the impression that the act had to be deliberate in order for it to be considered malpractice."

"How could a guy be so bad?" one student asked.

"Well, obviously," another student piped up, "he didn't know his anatomy."

"Or forgot what he had learned," I said. "Also, there was a rumor floating around that he may have been impaired." I could see that the students didn't know what I was talking about.

"Out to lunch," I said. "Drunk or stoned as the result of substance abuse. Do you people have any idea of how many surgeons are impaired? The latest estimate I've seen is about 15 percent. So take it easy on the weekends. You don't want to become that kind of a doctor. You could ruin a lot of lives."

"OKAY," I TOLD THEM. "That's enough of that. Let's get back to where we were in our thyroidectomy. We had made our incisions, lifted the strap muscles off the thyroid gland, and identified the recurrent laryngeal nerve in the groove between the trachea and the esophagus – and we're going to be extra careful not to cut or injure them, right?

"So now we're involved in gaining control of the arteries and the remaining veins going into and out of the thyroid gland. What are those vessels?"

"The superior and inferior thyroid arteries and veins."

"And what else?"

"The thyroid Ima artery," one of the A+ students replied. "It's seen in approximately ten percent of individuals."

"Very good," I said. I called on some slower students. "Show me the superior and inferior artery and veins." The first student did so. The second demonstrated the inferior thyroid veins and the third demonstrated the inferior thyroid arteries.

"Okay," I said, "what other structures could be damaged or removed by mistake during thyroidectomy? Nobody knows? Well, somebody show me a parathyroid gland."

One of the more reticent students pointed into the cadaver's neck. "Is this it, here?"

"Could be," I said. "It's in the right location. But it could be just fat or a lymph node. You'd need a microscopic exam to make sure it's parathyroid. Do you know how many of these glands there are?"

"Four."

"Always?" I asked. There were no answers, so I continued. "Eighty percent of us have four parathyroid glands. The rest of us – about 20% of us – have two, three, five or six. Now, how many of these glands can be removed without harming the patient?"

Even the A+ students were at a loss.

"Actually," I said, "no matter how many parathyroid glands we start out with, we need only one-half of one gland for normal calcium metabolism."

"What happens if all of them are damaged?"

"A really terrible condition called *hypoparathyroidism*. And, yes, I know of such a case. But we don't have the time to explore it right now. I'll get to it later. First, tell me what else can be damaged during ligation of the superior thyroid vessels?"

"The superior laryngeal nerve."

"Which branch?" I asked.

"The external branch," said the student, pointing to it.

"What does the nerve do?"

"It controls the crico-thyroid muscle."

I called on another student. "Show me that muscle," I said to her, "and tell me what the muscle does."

"It's right here," she said, "and it tenses the vocal cords."

"That's right. It's responsible for the high tones and the durability of the voice. Most of us might not miss this nerve or this muscle. But it is extremely important for people who lecture or speak a lot.

"Without this nerve, the voice fatigues easily. And, for a singer, the loss of this nerve or muscle is a disaster. Look closely: this tiny nerve is very, very close to the superior thyroid vessels in over 75%

of the cases you'll encounter. So the vessels need to be ligated as close to the thyroid as possible to avoid injury to that nerve.

"Surgeons call it the Galli-Curci nerve. The nerve was named for one of the greatest coloratura sopranos of all time. I have some of her recordings and she had a truly magnificent voice. It was stilled by a surgical mistake that could have been avoided.

"In 1935, Amelita Galli-Curci had developed a large goiter that was compressing her trachea and had to be removed. In the process, her superior laryngeal nerve was cut or damaged.

"Several months after her operation, she returned to the Chicago Opera House singing the role of Mimi in 'La Boheme.' But as the opera progressed, her upper range crumbled and her voice gave way to fatigue. Galli-Curci's brilliant career was over and, that night, the critics wrote obituaries for a legendary operatic voice."

"That's *so* sad," a young woman sighed.

"Very sad, and it didn't have to happen. It's been suggested that surgeons listen to operatic arias during thyroid operations so they'll remember to be extremely careful when ligating superior thyroid vessels."

I returned to the cadaver to finish the thyroidectomy instruction. "Once the blood supply to the gland has been interrupted, the thyroid gland can be totally removed. Of course, in a case like Galli-Curci's, only 90% of the gland would be removed. That would leave a portion of one lobe with its arterial supply intact."

"Do you know of any cases where the parathyroid glands were totally removed, Dr. Kessler?"

"Sure," I said. "Let me tell you about one of them. It happened here in the eastern United States. A famous head and neck surgeon accidentally cut the external branch of the superior laryngeal nerve."

"The Galli-Curci nerve," said one of the students.

"One and the same. But in this case it didn't belong to a world famous operatic diva, but to a healthy teenage girl who sang in her church choir. Following surgery, she could no longer sing. Her voice fatigued easily and it crackled if she talked a lot.

"The injury to her vocal mechanism was unfortunate, but it was really the least of her problems. The girl had undergone neck exploration twice for the removal of overactive parathyroid glands.

"As you've seen, there are usually four such tiny glands behind or below the thyroid gland and they control calcium metabolism. If one or all of these glands becomes overactive, the calcium level becomes too high and that can cause death. So, when removing the offending gland or glands, it's important to leave behind at least one half of a single parathyroid gland.

"If all the glands are removed, the calcium level becomes too low and that can cause a serious derangement in calcium metabolism with dire consequences. That is to say, removing all the glands can be life threatening.

"Now, during surgical exploration, it can be difficult to identify a parathyroid gland. It can look like a piece of fat or a lymph node. So it's imperative to obtain a tiny biopsy of all tissue you think *might* be parathyroid gland.

"The small biopsy should be examined immediately by a pathologist who can determine if the specimen is parathyroid gland or not. That should be done *before* any gland or tissue is totally removed.

"During the second exploration of this teenager's neck, her surgeon removed over 15 specimens of tissue, but he failed to get an immediate pathological exam (frozen section) in over half of them.

"It was only *after* the operation that a pathological examination of all the tissue specimens showed that the surgeon had removed all four of the teenager's parathyroid glands. So, now the girl has permanent hypoparathyroidism with frequent episodes of low calcium levels. That causes tetany – muscle spasm – plus numbness around the mouth and facial grimacing. She also has trouble breathing.

"This sort of metabolic derangement is difficult to control with medication such as calcium or Vitamin D. Patients can also experience mood swings, brittle finger nails, defective teeth, loss of hair (including eyebrows), cataracts and calcifications in the arteries and the brain. When calcium levels become dangerously low, patients have to rush to the emergency room to get calcium intravenously.

"This teenage girl's disability is permanent. Her surgeon deviated from the accepted standards of parathyroid surgery by failing to get tissue removed for frozen sections. As a result, he removed all the glands without knowing it."

"I hope he was sued," one of the students said. "He was, wasn't he?"

"He was, but it wasn't easy for the girl's attorney to pursue this case. No head and neck expert in that metropolitan area was willing to testify against a surgeon who had written textbooks on the subject. The girl's lawyer had to go to a different part of the country to get the surgical and pathological experts he needed. But he did get them and, in the end, the defendant settled out of court. I don't know how much money was involved, but I hope the sum was large."

None of the students seemed to be in a hurry to leave, so I told them about another doctor who should have known better: a surgeon who had performed hundreds of parathyroidectomies during his career. Even so, he removed two large parathyroid glands, one on each side of his patient's neck.

"Following surgery, the patient developed hypoparathyroidism. The pathology report revealed that the glands he had removed were normal glands – no tumor, no hyperplasia. The surgeon had not obtained a biopsy of any of the tissue. But he claimed that he had left two parathyroid glands on the anterior aspect of the thyroid. "

The students asked if the patient had died. "Yes," I told them, "but from a bad heart. The post-op hypoparathyroidism may have pushed him over the edge. That's just my opinion, not a fact.

"But, here's what's interesting. At autopsy, no remaining parathyroid tissue could be found. What the surgeon was dealing with was a rare case of an embryonic abnormality where four glands had fused into two."

"Why didn't the surgeon get a small biopsy before removing the glands?"

"Because he was arrogant," I said. "Some surgeons get so cocky that they believe they can identify a parathyroid gland with their naked eyeball 100% of the time. Well, that's just not so. In both of the cases I've told you about, the surgeons got into trouble because of arrogance."

I was about to let my students hustle off to begin cramming for the final exam, but I saw that one young man had his hand raised.

"My Mom had a disc operation on her neck, Dr. Kessler. You know, the cervical spine? They cut her recurrent laryngeal nerve, like you were telling us about."

There was dead silence for several moments. Students from a nearby table left their cadaver and gathered around. I asked my student if his Mom had a history of neck problems.

"Nothing that required surgery," he said. "Not until this time."

"This is not supposed to happen in a neck that's never been operated on. There's no scar tissue or inflammation to make the dissection difficult or hazardous. There's no excuse for making this kind of surgical mistake."

"I was pretty sure that someone screwed up," the young man said. "Now they're planning a nerve bypass or something like that. What do you think my Mom should do?"

"I'd need to examine her and study her surgeon's treatment plan in detail before venturing a medical opinion. But I can tell this much right now. Your Mom should get a second opinion from *somebody*." As he left, I added: "And she should get a damn good lawyer!"

Had that last remark been necessary? Had I been too blunt? It was the poor kid's first year in medical school, after all, and he'd already been given a lot more information than he'd bargained for. But he and his classmates had every right to be told the truth, awful as it might be, so they could learn from it.

EVERYONE WAS GONE NOW – the students and the two other instructors. The anatomy laboratory was silent, as still as death. I was alone with my thoughts, just me and my 26 cadavers.

I'd managed to avoid looking at all of them before the students arrived that morning, but I couldn't put it off any longer. I walked slowly back across the room toward Table 9 and the cadaver I had been avoiding all semester. Slowly, I removed the head covering and looked at Joe's face.

I've never been sentimental about cadavers, but I had found Joe's presence in my lab unsettling. Was it because we were the same age? Was I shocked by the sudden reminder of my own mortality? Perhaps.

As I looked down at his white hair and waxy brown skull, an Irish ballad came to mind: "*The roses all have left her cheeks; I watched them fade away and die . . . .*" His cheeks too, I thought. And his friendly smile, as well.

Joe's face was still intact, but it was expressionless. His feet extended beyond the edge of the table and the rest of him had been dissected all the way up into his neck. Even so, there was enough of him left for the final exam.

"Well, Joe," I said, "you've got another week before you retire." I spoke quietly, on the off chance that his spirit was someplace where he could hear my voice or read my mind.

"I told you often how we learn from the dead here. It looks like my students learned a lot from you. Pretty soon, the final exam will be over and you'll be able to rest in peace, my friend. You've done valuable service here, Joe."

I zipped up his head covering and whispered, "Thank you, Joe."

THE FINAL ANATOMY EXAMINATION went off without a hitch. All my students passed and moved on.

When I next visited the anatomy lab, all the tables were empty. Joe's cadaver was gone and so were the cadavers of all the other generous people who had helped teach anatomy to the living – and helped me show another class of first-year medical students how to "Do no harm" when they became physicians.

The End

AFTERWORD

▬▬

NOW THAT YOU'VE HAD A CHANCE to learn something about my credentials and evaluate my credibility, you can ponder what I've presented and make up your own mind about controversial issues in the current public discourse about health care in the United States. That's your job, not mine. My hope is that some of the points I've tried to make (and some of the opinions I've expressed) will help you come to your own conclusions.

Something I hope you bear in mind is that medical malpractice is a reality – and it's not caused by lawyers. "Tort reform" will not make it go away.

Mistakes happen. Most surgical errors or accidents can be corrected in the operating room before the patient is closed up. And any good surgeon would do just that: repair the damage immediately. But, as you've seen, that's not always what happens.

Several years ago, just to satisfy my own curiosity, I took a second look at 45 cases I had recently reviewed for attorneys. All 45 had resulted in serious disabilities or death. I found that every one of those bad outcomes was the result of an avoidable technical error. What struck me was that in a full 75% of those cases, the technical errors had not been recognized at the time they were made. If any of the surgeons had been aware of the accidental injuries and had repaired the damage right away, no lasting harm would have been done in most of those cases. Instead, their patients were disabled – or died.

Over the years, there have been amazing technological advances in the practice of medicine. Improvements in CT scans, MRIs, PET scans and ultra-sound techniques have greatly enhanced physicians' diagnostic abilities. Endoscopic surgery has been perfected so rapidly that these tools are now used in a variety of sub-specialties including head-and-neck, cardiac and vascular surgery. Abdominal surgeons are now performing major procedures with the aid of fiber-optic endoscopes thus decreasing post-operative pain and the length of hospital stays. All well and good.

But could advances in medical technology eventually make medical malpractice a thing of the past? Don't hold your breath. I'm afraid that advanced technology will have little impact on the incidence of medical malpractice events. The cases I've presented in this book reveal a recurring deficiency that cannot be changed by modern technology.

Think about the errors you've examined: failure to go to a patients bedside when a critical situation demands it; failure to obtain a consultation with another physician in a timely manner; procrastination in the diagnostic work-up of patients who may have cancer; excessive use of narcotics and other sedatives before a diagnosis has been established; inappropriate use of antibiotics; managing critical patients primarily by telephone. No, I doubt that advances in technology will end medical malpractice incidents, unless some genius invents a machine that can change human nature. Or, failing that, at least develops a vaccine for some of the Seven Deadly Sins that you've observed running rampant through these pages.

Also, while reading this book, you probably became aware of the many bad outcomes caused by ignorance or forgetfulness about certain parts of the body – surgeons inadvertently cutting that Galli-Curci nerve, for example, because they didn't know (or just forgot) that it was there.

Human anatomy is one of the most important subjects a future doctor must study. It always has been and always will be. But it's just one of the basic sciences medical students spend most of their time studying during the early years of their training. And gradually over the years, the time spent on the study of human anatomy has been decreased to make room for subjects that didn't even exist when I was a student: genetics and cellular biology, for example.

When I first studied anatomy with Dr. Grant, it was a 400 hour course. Today, some medical schools have cut the time spent studying the gross anatomy of the human body to less than 90 hours. In my opinion, that's cutting too deep.

Also, in an effort to manage time and control costs, some medical schools have abolished cadaver dissection in favor of anatomical models. These life-like models can be useful adjuncts, but they should *never* replace cadavers. When it comes to human beings, one size does not fit all. Your appendix, for example, may not be on the same side of the body as mine is, so I should not assume that your abdominal pain is *not* caused by appendicitis. That's something I learned in the anatomy lab years ago.

While I disagree with the administrative decisions regarding anatomy courses, I understand why such decisions have to be made. There is much more than anatomy for modern medical students to learn and only so much time in which to learn it. But students learn many important things from the dead, as you have read, not all of them scientific: compassion, humility and awareness of their own mortality. By reducing the time they are allowed to contemplate their cadavers, I fear we risk creating a generation of robotic physicians who may do serious harm to their patients because their knowledge of anatomy – and humanity – is deficient.

Could that be symptomatic of a high price we will all have to pay for rapid technical and scientific progress – the hidden cost of the explosion of knowledge and expertise? Will we be able to perform complex tasks even faster, but have less and less time for listening and learning and understanding? Will that be true for everybody, not just those of us in the medical profession? Will we be unable to make good decisions because there will be far too much to decide?

Perhaps not. The young people in my anatomy lab this past semester were just as motivated and idealistic as those who came before. There was less time to tell my stories, but I got the same reactions to the ones I did tell them. Unlike my 20th Century students, they texted and Tweeted and typed their notes with their thumbs! Amazing!

I'm pretty sure that my young 21st Century students – and other young people who come after them – will diagnose what's wrong with American health care, fix it and make it better for everybody. They seem to want to do that. And I hope my stories will help.

Oh, yeah. A note for today's doctors, nurses, technicians and administrators about how to avoid malpractice lawsuits: "Do no harm."

And, for those who still don't get it: "Physician, heal thyself."

ABOUT THE AUTHORS

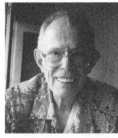

RICHARD KESSLER, M.D., F.A.C.S., retired from the practice of medicine in 1995 after more than 30 years as a surgeon at the VA Hospital in Manhattan. He was also an attending surgeon at Bellevue Hospital. As a full professor at the NYU Medical School, he taught surgery and anatomy.

After college, Dick Kessler spent a post-graduate year studying anatomy at the University of Toronto with Dr. J.C. Boileau Grant, a leading 20th Century anatomist, whose *Grant's Atlas of Anatomy* is still a required text book. Upon entering McGill University's medical school in Montreal, he was asked to teach the first-year anatomy course because of his 400 hours of instruction from Dr. Grant. At this writing, he is still teaching anatomy to first-year medical students at NYU.

Dr. Kessler has published 60 articles and abstracts in peer review journals, but he wanted this book to be readable for people with no medical training. "Because of the confusion caused by the debate about health care reform," he told his co-author, "I feel an obligation to tell what I have seen, heard, and learned first-hand over half-a-century as a medical student, an intern, a resident, a practicing physician, general surgeon, U.S. Army doctor, teacher, researcher and expert witness in medical malpractice law suits."

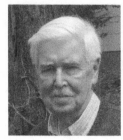 PATRICK TRESE, an original staff member of the Huntley-Brinkley Report, has been writing professionally since his senior year in college, mostly network news and documentaries for NBC News where he learned to translate complicated legal, political and scientific language into plain, readable English.

His book about making documentary films in Antarctica in 1957-58, *Penguins Have Square Eyes,* was published by Holt, Rinehart & Winston in 1962. *Caril,* the story of Caril Ann Fugate, who became involved with mass-murderer Charles Starkweather and was convicted of first degree murder at age 15, was published by Lippincott in 1972. It was based on his NBC News investigative documentary "Growing Up in Prison."

During his 30 years at NBC, his awards included a Peabody and several Emmys. After retirement, he wrote the 10-part PBS series "America Goes to War," narrated by Eric Sevareid and 12 episodes of "The 20th Century" series narrated by Mike Wallace for CBS News Productions. He will soon publish his novel, *AMDG: An Ignatian Thriller.*